NUCLEAR RECEPTORS AS MOLECULAR TARGETS FOR CARDIOMETABOLIC AND CENTRAL NERVOUS SYSTEM DISEASES

Solvay Pharmaceuticals Conferences

Series Editors

Werner Cautreels, Claus Steinborn and Lechoslaw Turski

Volume 8

Previously published in this series

ISSN 1566-7685

Nuclear Receptors as Molecular Targets for Cardiometabolic and Central Nervous System Diseases

Edited by

J.L. Junien

Laboratoires Fournier, a Solvay Pharmaceuticals company, Daix, France

and

B. Staels

Inserm U.545, Institut Pasteur de Lille, Lille, France

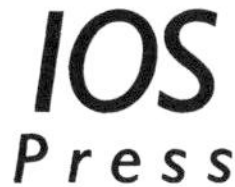

Press

Amsterdam • Berlin • Oxford • Tokyo • Washington, DC

ISBN 978-1-58603-857-1
Library of Congress Control Number: 2008925578

Publisher
IOS Press
Nieuwe Hemweg 6B
1013 BG Amsterdam
Netherlands
fax: +31 20 687 0019
e-mail: order@iospress.nl

Distributor in the UK and Ireland
Gazelle Books Services Ltd.
White Cross Mills
Hightown
Lancaster LA1 4XS
United Kingdom
fax: +44 1524 63232
e-mail: sales@gazellebooks.co.uk

Distributor in the USA and Canada
IOS Press, Inc.
4502 Rachael Manor Drive
Fairfax, VA 22032
USA
fax: +1 703 323 3668
e-mail: iosbooks@iospress.com

Preface

**"The Solvay Pharmaceuticals Conferences:
where industry meets academia in a search for novel therapies"**

Nuclear Receptors Take Off

The cloning of the first nuclear receptor cDNA encoding the human glucocorticoid receptor was described in 1985 by the team of Evans [1]. Over the next 25 years a dramatic growth of knowledge on nuclear receptors followed this discovery [2]. The knowledge on nuclear receptors has delivered novel therapies for lipid control and hormone replacement, and for management of cancers and diabetes, and millions of humans were subjected to therapies with nuclear receptor modulators over last decades [2,3].

Nuclear receptors are a family of transcription factors consisting of 49 members identified in the human genome [3]. Nuclear receptors regulate transcription by binding to response elements in the regulatory regions of target genes and thereby affect expression of genes involved in differentiation, growth, lipid homeostasis, inflammation and immunity. Therefore, nuclear receptors are attractive molecular targets for design of therapy for diabetes, obesity, atherosclerosis, cancer, inflammation and neurodegeneration.

Many drugs from the armamentarium of contemporary physicians are acting on nuclear receptors: estrogens for hormone replacement therapy, anti-estrogens for treatment of cancer, steroids for treatment of inflammatory disorders, fibrates for treatment of dyslipidemia, and thiazolidinediones for therapy of diabetes [2].

Through their distinct tissue distribution and specific target gene activation, the peroxisome proliferator-activated receptors (PPARs) α, γ and δ modulate diverse aspects of fatty acid metabolism, energy balance, insulin sensitivity, glucose homeostasis and inflammatory responses. Two types of PPARs are marketed: PPARα is the target for fibrates (hypolipidemic drugs), PPARγ is the target for thiazolidinediones (anti-diabetic drugs).

The Liver X Receptors (LXRs) modulate macrophage cholesterol efflux and repress the expression of pro-inflammatory genes. Therefore, LXRs are considered as a target for the treatment of atherosclerosis (prevention and reversal). LXRs are key players in inflammatory conditions such as rheumatoid arthritis, inflammatory bowel diseases and diabetes. Through action on both cholesterol homeostasis and inflammatory processes, LXRs are considered as prospective targets for design of novel therapies for Alzheimer's disease.

Thyroid hormone signals are transduced by two distinct nuclear receptors: TRα and TRβ. TRα mediates the effects of thyroid hormones on heart rate whereas TRβ mediates cholesterol lowering effects. Therapeutic use of these receptors has not substantiated yet, but both are carefully considered by drug developers.

In addition to transcriptional regulation of metabolic pathways, nuclear receptors regulate the expression of genes participating in inflammatory cascades as well as genes promoting cellular growth and differentiation. Therefore, nuclear receptors continue to be important for the development of novel therapies of inflammation, cancer and neurodegeneration.

This volume contains papers from the Eight Solvay Pharmaceuticals Conference on Nuclear Receptors as Molecular Targets for Cardiometabolic and Central Nervous System Diseases held in Nice (France) April 11–13, 2007.

It has been the aim of these conferences to bring together scientists from academia and from industry in order to stimulate dialog between them in a congenial setting. The focus of this conference centered on the mechanistic involvement of nuclear receptors in cardiological, metabolic and neurological disorders, on possible explanation of pathways involved in pathogenesis, on susceptibility to and prevention of metabolic and neurological disorders and on the aspects of drug finding including chemistry and rational drug design. New technologies were highlighted including gene expression, novel approaches towards epigenetics, physiological monitoring and prospective use of novel therapeutics.

W. Cautreels
C. Steinborn
L. Turski

References

[1] S.M. Hollenberg, C. Weinberger C, E.S. Ong *et al.* Primary structure and expression of a functional human glucocorticoid receptor cDNA. *Nature* **318** (1985) 635-641.
[2] R.M. Evans. The nuclear receptor superfamily: a rosetta stone for physiology. *Mol. Endocrinol.* **19** (2005) 1429-1438.
[3] D.L. Morganstein and M.G. Parker. Role of nuclear receptor coregulators in metabolism. *Exp. Rev. Endocrinol. Metab.* **2** (2007) 797-807.

List of Contributors

Cautreels, W.
Solvay Pharmaceuticals, Brussels, Belgium

Duez, H.
Inserm U.545, Institut Pasteur de Lille, 1 rue du Professeur Calmette, BP 245, 59019
Lille, France; and Université de Lille 2, Lille, 59006 France

Edwards, P.A.
Department of Biological Chemistry, University of California at Los Angeles, 33-257
CHS, 10833 Le Conte Ave., Los Angeles, CA 90095, USA
Department of Medicine, University of California at Los Angeles, 33-257 CHS, 10833
Le Conte Ave., Los Angeles, CA 90095, USA
The Molecular Biology Institute, University of California at Los Angeles, CA 90095,
USA

Giguère, V.
McGill University Health Centre, 687 Pine Avenue West, Montréal, Québec, H3A 1A1,
Canada

Häring, H.-U.
Department of Internal Medicine, Division of Endocrinology, Diabetology, Angiology,
Nephrology, and Clinical Chemistry, Eberhard-Karls-University Tübingen, Otfried-
Müller-Strasse 10, 72076 Tübingen, Germany

Heneka, M.T.
Department of Neurology, Molecular Neurology Unit, University of Münster, Albert
Schweitzer-Strasse 33, 48149 Münster, Germany

Junien, J.L.
Laboratoires Fournier, a Solvay Pharmaceuticals company, 50 rue de Dijon, 21121
Daix, France

Kuipers, F.
Laboratory of Pediatrics, Center for Liver, Digestive, and Metabolic Diseases, University Medical Center Groningen, Hanzeplein 1, 9700 RB Groningen, The Netherlands

Laudet, V.
Molecular Zoology, Institut de Génomique Fonctionelle de Lyon; UMR 5242 du
CNRS; INRA; IFR128 BioSciences Lyon-Gerland; Université de Lyon; Ecole Normale
Supérieure de Lyon, 46 Allée d'Italie, 69364 Lyon Cedex 07, France

viii

Mulder, M.
Department of Basic Neurosciences, Institute Brain & Behavior, EURON, Maastricht University, Universiteitssingel 50, 6229 ER Maastricht, The Netherlands

Paxian, S.A.
Department of Neurology, Molecular Neurology Unit, University of Münster, Albert Schweitzer-Strasse 33, 48149 Münster, Germany

Staels, B.
Inserm U.545, Institut Pasteur de Lille, 1 rue du Professeur Calmette, BP 245, 59019 Lille, France; and Université de Lille 2, Lille, 59006 France

Staiger, H.
Department of Internal Medicine, Division of Endocrinology, Diabetology, Angiology, Nephrology, and Clinical Chemistry, Eberhard-Karls-University Tübingen, Otfried-Müller-Strasse 10, 72076 Tübingen, Germany

Steinborn,C.
Solvay Pharmaceuticals, Hannover, Germany

Tatenhorst, L.
Department of Neurology, Molecular Neurology Unit, University of Münster, Albert Schweitzer-Strasse 33, 48149 Münster, Germany

Thamer, C.
Department of Internal Medicine, Division of Endocrinology, Diabetology, Angiology, Nephrology, and Clinical Chemistry, Eberhard-Karls-University Tübingen, Otfried-Müller-Strasse 10, 72076 Tübingen, Germany

Tiel, C.M. van
Department of Medical Biochemistry, Academic Medical Center, University of Amsterdam, Meibergdreef 15, 1105 AZ Amsterdam, The Netherlands

Turski, L.
Solvay Pharmaceuticals, Weesp, The Netherlands

Vries, C.J.M. de
Department of Medical Biochemistry, Academic Medical Center, University of Amsterdam, Meibergdreef 15, 1105 AZ Amsterdam, The Netherlands

Zhang, Y.
Department of Biological Chemistry, University of California at Los Angeles, 33-257 CHS, 10833 Le Conte Ave., Los Angeles, CA 90095, USA
Department of Medicine, University of California at Los Angeles, 33-257 CHS, 10833 Le Conte Ave., Los Angeles, CA 90095, USA

Contents

Conference Preface
and
Keynote Lecture

Conference Preface

Nuclear Receptors (NRs) are transcription factors, which control pathways that may be modified in pathological conditions, by regulating the expression of genes. The NR superfamily is composed of several subfamilies, with common characteristics in terms of structure, mode of activation and gene regulation, which makes this family attractive for researchers from both Academy and Pharmaceutical Industry to study their physiological functions and to decipher their potential as new targets for specific diseases.

The NR field has been one of the most successful research areas for the pharmaceutical industry, having yielded not only breakthrough drugs for serious diseases, such as immuno-inflammation, cancer, endocrinology, metabolic diseases, but also a high number of drugs per target (e.g. glucocorticoids, steroid hormones, mineralocorticoids, retinoids, fibrates and glitazones).

Interestingly, the NR family remains relatively little exploited, since, among the 48 members of this family in man, only few receptors have been extensively investigated. There is therefore a clear need to better understand these "new" receptors, in terms of their structure, how they function, what their endogenous ligands, if any, are, what their role in physiological and pathological conditions are, which diseases they modulate and what the potential risks associated with new drugs acting on these receptors are. It is known for long that NRs play a central role in the peripheral control of metabolic homeostasis, but more and more evidence indicates a role also in the brain where they control not only metabolic and inflammatory pathways, but also indirectly the neuronal machinery.

Nowadays, a major challenge is to move from symptomatic treatment to curative or preventive therapies, and new knowledge, technologies and paradigms have to be developed and applied to modern drug discovery. For instance, as the pathophysiological mechanisms in Alzheimer's disease are becoming better understood, modulatory roles for a number of NRs, such as the LXRs or PPARs, have been reported.

NRs appear more difficult targets than, for instance, membrane receptors, since they reside inside the cell, act in the nucleus and control several pathways. However, NRs have the potential to impact on serious diseases and the benefit/risk has always to be assessed as early as possible, at preclinical and clinical stages, and put in perspective with other proposed therapies.

It is our belief that the therapeutic potential of each nuclear receptor is vast. This is nicely illustrated in this meeting's proceedings for the LXRs, FXR, PPARs and NURRs which have existing or potential pharmacological applications for the treatment not only of cardiometabolic diseases but also CNS disorders.

Bart Staels   Jean Louis Junien

IOS Press, 2008

An Introduction to the Nuclear Receptor Superfamily

Vincent Laudet

Molecular Zoology, Institut de Génomique Fonctionelle de Lyon;
UMR 5242 du CNRS; INRA; IFR128 BioSciences Lyon-Gerland; Université de Lyon;
Ecole Normale Supérieure de Lyon, 46 Allée d'Italie, 69364 Lyon Cedex 07, France

Abstract. Nuclear receptors (NRs) are major targets for drug discovery and play key roles in development and homeostasis, as well as in many diseases such as obesity, diabetes and cancer. This review provides a general overview of the mechanism of action of nuclear receptors and explores the various factors that are instrumental in modulating their pharmacology. One of the most promising aspects of nuclear receptor pharmacology is that it is now possible to develop ligands with a large spectrum of full, partial or inverse agonist or antagonist activities, but also compounds, called selective nuclear receptor modulators, that activate only a subset of the functions induced by the cognate ligand or that act in a cell-type-selective manner.

Keywords. Nuclear Receptors, orphan receptors, ligands, evolution, SERMs

Introduction

Many hydrophobic hormones such as estrogens, thyroid hormones, and corticoids, but also food-derived compounds such as fatty acid and cholesterol metabolites play important roles in physiological processes including reproduction, homeostasis control and embryonic development [1]. Each of these hormones can be implicated in a wide array of effects in a single organism. For example, estrogens, in addition to their critical role in reproduction, have been implicated in reducing the incidence of coronary heart disease and in maintaining bone mineral density (reviewed in [2]). However, the use of estrogens is also associated with an increased risk of uterine and breast cancer, factors which limit their use by many postmenopausal women. In addition, the actions of estrogens are mimicked by a variety of xenoestrogenic compounds including synthetic steroids, pesticides, industrial chemicals and phytoestrogens leading to potentially adverse health effects in humans and wildlife [3].

The actions of these hydrophobic hormones within the organism are mediated through a conserved family of ligand-activated transcription factors, the nuclear receptor (NR) superfamily which consists of 48 genes in human [1]. Because of the essential role played by NRs in virtually all aspects of mammalian development, metabolism and physiology, dysfunctions of signalling pathways controlled by these receptors are associated with reproductive, proliferative and metabolic diseases [1,4]. The ligand-binding ability of half of the nuclear receptors makes them promising pharmaceutical targets. Every liganded NR has one or more cognate natural or synthetic ligands that are used in therapy. Classical examples include retinoic acid targeting RARα in acute promyelocytic leukaemia, the synthetic ERα antagonist tamoxifen used in the treatment of breast cancer, dexamethasone for GR (used in the treatment of inflammatory diseases), and thiazolidinediones that are a treatment for type-2 diabetes and bind PPARγ [4]. Interest in developing NR-targeting drugs has been reinforced recently by the realization that it would be possible to generate compounds collectively referred to as SNuRMs (Selective Nuclear Receptor Modulators) that may have tissue-specific effects (i.e. that may behave as agonists in some tissues while behaving as antagonists in others) and/or promoter specific effects (i.e. that may regulate only certain genes and not others) [4-6].

This short review will describe in general terms the structure and mode of action of nuclear receptors. It will also discuss NR ligands, an apparently simple concept that has considerably evolved over the years. Through the knowledge on NR ligand mode of action, this review will show what the main trends are to explain the specificity behind SNuRM action.

1. The Superfamily

Let's start by presenting in general terms the main actors of the drama. The NR superfamily includes receptors for hydrophobic molecules such as steroid hormones (e.g. estrogens, glucocorticoids, progesterone, mineralocorticoids, androgens, vitamin D, oxysterols, bile acids and ecdysteroids in insects), retinoic acids (all-*trans* and 9-*cis* isoforms, although the *in vivo* relevance of 9-*cis* retinoic acid is strongly debated), thyroid hormones, fatty acids, leukotrienes and prostaglandins [4]. NRs are known in all metazoan phyla but are still not known in other organisms (e.g. plants, fungi or unicellular eukaryotes) although some distantly NR-related sequences were recently described in fungi [7,8]. The number of NR genes varies widely from one organism to another: 48 in human, 49 in mouse, 71 in zebrafish (fish have duplicated their genome a long time ago), 21 in Drosophila and more than 270 in the nematode *C. elegans* in which massive duplication of a unique NR, HNF4 has occurred [9,10]. Overall and despite species variations and strikingly bizarre situations (such as the case of a NR with 2 DBDs recently described in a flatworm, *Schistosoma* [11]), one should retain that there are classically ca. 45-50 NR genes in vertebrates and ca. 18-20 in invertebrates [9].

All NRs share several conserved functional domains such as the DNA-binding domain (DBD) and the ligand-binding domain (LBD). In fact, in the final years of the last century, many NRs have been identified through their sequence identity with these conserved domains since the original cloning of the first members of the superfamily (ERα and GR) [1]. Strikingly, several of these newly identified have no identified natural ligand and are referred to as «orphan receptors». It is still unknown whether these orphan receptors are classical, liganded receptors with ligands that remain to be discovered or if they are real orphans (i.e. constitutively active transcriptional regulators whose activity can be regulated by other mechanisms). Among these orphan receptors, some are clearly real orphans because they do not contain the domain implicated in ligand binding. This is the case for example of the Drosophila genes KNI, KNRL and EAGLE, and several nematode NR genes. Notably, other receptors, such as the DAX-1 gene implicated in sex determination in vertebrates and its paralogue SHP, which is important for cholesterol homeostasis, have a complementary structure because they contain a ligand-binding domain (LBD) but no classical DNA-binding domain (DBD) (reviewed in [1]) (What about NR4A??). Although ligands have since been described for several orphan receptors such as LXR, FXR, PXR and CAR, the identity of the ligands, if any, of other orphan receptors such as COUP-TFI or TLL is still a mystery. In fact, among the 48 known NRs in the human genome, only 24 are clearly liganded receptors, (even if the definition of a liganded receptor will be dependent of our definition of a ligand).

The existence of orphan receptors raises some interesting questions regarding their origin and relationship with liganded receptors. In fact, the evolutionary origin of the NR family is still marred with the controversy of whether the ancestral receptor was a liganded or an orphan receptor. For the latter scenario, regulation of NR activity through ligand binding would have to have evolved several times independently [7,10,12].

Owing to the multitude of different names given to NR gene products, an official nomenclature was proposed by the Nuclear Receptor Nomenclature Committee in 1999 [13] that relies on the phylogenetic relationships of the receptors. Indeed, sequence alignment and phylogenetic tree construction resulted in the classification of the human NR family into seven evolutionary groups of unequal size [7,13]. A correlation exists between the DNA-binding and dimerization abilities of each NR and its phylogenetic position. This is not the case for ligand-binding ability; an observation that favours a model of independent gain of ligand binding during evolution, starting from an ancestral orphan receptor (Figure 1):

1. This large group contains the TRs, RARs, VDR and PPARs, as well as orphan receptors such as the RORs, Rev-erbs, CAR (NR1I3), PXR (NR1I2), LXRs, etc.
2. This group includes RXRs, COUP-TF and HNF4.
3. This group includes the steroid receptors such as ERs, GR, PR, AR, as well as the ERRs.
4. This small group contains the NGFI-B group of orphan receptors (NGFI-B (NR4A1), Nurr1 (NR4A2), NOR-1 (NR4A3)).
5. This is another small group that includes SF-1 (NR5A1) and the receptors related to the *Drosophila* FTZ-F1.
6. This subgroup consists solely of the GCNF1 receptor (NR6A1), which does not fit well into any other subgroups.
7. The receptors with a conserved domain (either LBD or DBD) missing such as the DAX-1 and SHP receptors are arbitrarily clustered into a seventh subfamily, called NR0

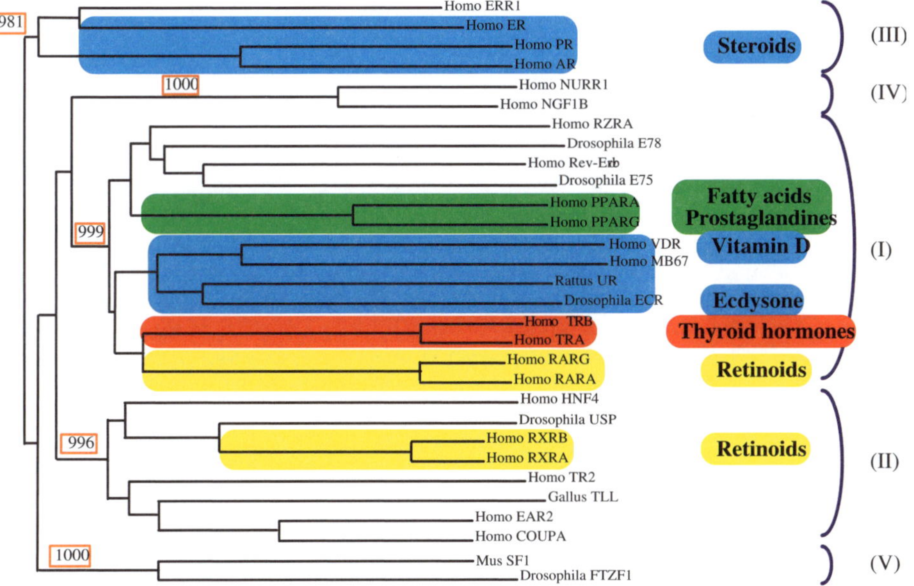

Figure 1. A phylogeny of the nuclear receptor superfamily highlighting the 7 major subfamilies. The robustness value supporting each subfamily branch is boxed in red. The chemical nature of the ligand is indicated by a colour code. Orphan receptors are in white.

2. Nuclear Receptors for Beginners

Nuclear receptors are modular proteins, possessing several domains that carry out specific functions required for their activities as ligand-regulated transcription factors. Most NRs bear an N-terminal ligand-independent transcriptional activation domain (AF-1), a centrally located DNA-binding domain (DBD) consisting of a strongly conserved core region of 66 amino-acids which encodes for two zinc finger modules, a flexible hinge that allows flexibility between the N- and C-terminal part of the molecule, and a C-terminal ligand-binding domain (LBD), which interacts with the ligand, allows receptor dimerization and additionally serves as a ligand-activated transcriptional activation function (AF-2). Following ligand binding, the ligand-binding domain undergoes a conformational change during which the most C-terminal helix, H12, forms a lid that closes the hydrophobic pocket in which the ligand is buried (reviewed in [6,14]). It has been shown that this conformational change triggers a major shift in the co-regulatory proteins (co-repressors and co-activators) that are able to interact with the ligand-binding domain. This "mouse-trap" model is still basically correct but has been completed over the year: it is now clear that the LBD is in an equilibrium between these two conformations and that the ligand induces a shift in this equilibrium.

Nuclear receptors can bind to DNA either as monomers (for example, steroidogenic factor-1 SF-1), homodimers (for example, steroid receptors such as ER), or heterodimers with the promiscuous Retinoid X Receptor (RXR) (for example RAR, TR, VDR and several orphan receptors) [1]. Nuclear receptor response elements are derivatives of the canonical sequence PuGGTCA, called hormone response elements (HREs). Modification, extension and duplication (including alternate relative orientations of the repeat such as direct, inverted or everted) of this sequence generates response elements that are selective for a given receptor(s) or class of receptors (for example, estrogen response elements (EREs) for ERs or retinoic acid response elements, RARE for RAR-RXR; see [1] for a review). By binding as dimers to sequence-specific response elements located in the regulatory regions of their target genes nuclear receptors exert either positive or negative control over the rates of transcription.

Through these response elements but also via alternate mechanisms including cross-talk with other signalling pathways (e.g. AP-1, NFκB, STAT), NRs exert control over complex networks of genes that mediate various aspects of the action of their ligands [1], [15]. Given that most NR ligands have wide pleiotropic actions in the body these networks could be complex and variable from one organ to another but also from one physiological condition to another. For example, estrogens are key regulators of growth, differentiation, and the physiological functions of a wide range of target tissues including the male and female reproductive tracts, breast, and skeletal, nervous, cardiovascular, digestive and immune systems. In addition, estrogens are known to regulate cell proliferation in breast cancer cells and uterine endometrium [2,16-18]. Among the well-known direct targets of estrogens in breast that may explain their role in activating breast cancer cell proliferation, are the pS2 gene also known as TFF1 (trefoil factor 1) that exhibits complex regulation by estrogens and growth factors, the cathepsin D gene encoding a lysosomal proteinase, the c-myc proto-oncogene, various cyclin genes, the progesterone receptor gene, as well as another member of the nuclear receptor superfamily, the growth factor gene TGFα [16-18].

Numerous *in vitro* studies have shown that the LBD is a functionally complex and dynamic domain as it mediates ligand-binding, dimerization and contains a ligand-dependent transactivation function. The LBD contains three structurally distinct but functionally linked surfaces: (*i*) a dimerization surface, which mediates interaction with partner LBDs, e.g. RXR, (*ii*) the ligand-binding pocket (LBP), which interacts with the small lipophilic ligand (in the case of liganded NRs), (*iii*) a co-regulator binding surface, which binds to regulatory protein complexes that modulate transcriptional activity positively or negatively. Part of this surface corresponds to an activation function helix, termed AF-2, which mediates ligand-dependent transactivation [6,14,19]. Within AF-2, the integrity of a conserved amphipathic α-helix called helix 12 has been shown to be required for ligand-dependent transactivation and co-activator recruitment.

The first resolution of a NR LBD crystal structure, the unliganded RXRα, revealed that the LBD is a highly structured domain [20]. This crystal structure, together with the elucidation of the 3D-structures of multiple other nuclear receptor LBDs, showed a common fold comprising 10-13 α-helices (H) and a short β-turn (s1-s2), arranged in three layers to form an anti-parallel "α-helical sandwich". Helices H1-H3 constitute one face of the LBD ([21], reviewed in [14]). H4, H5, s1-s2, H8 and H9 correspond to the central layer of the domain and H6, H7 and H10 form the second face. The superposition of all available LBD structures reveals a clear overall similarity, particularly in the top half of the LBD, that includes H1, H4, H5 and H7-H10 and corresponds to a structurally rather invariable region. The lower part of the LBD harbours a variable region, which contains the ligand-binding pocket (LBP).

Their mode of activation has made nuclear receptors an attractive system in which to study the mechanisms of transcriptional regulation. Several different classes of proteins interact with NRs to enhance or inhibit their activity as *trans*-acting factors, and these interacting proteins include co-activators, co-integrators, co-repressors, and multiple proteins associated with the basal transcription machinery (reviewed in [22,23]). In the absence of hormone, many receptors actively repress transcription via direct interactions with co-repressors such as NCoR, SMRT or SunCoR. It was shown recently that a conserved motif in NCoR and SMRT, called the CoRNR box, interacts with a groove in the LBD surface that is topologically very similar but not identical to that recognized by co-activators ([1,4,6,19]). These co-repressors recruit high molecular weight complexes that display histone deacetylase activities. Deacetylated histones are associated with silent regions of the genome, and it is generally accepted that histone deacetylation shuffles nucleosomal targets toward a condensed chromatin configuration which leads to transcriptional repression. Although unliganded estrogen receptors do not repress transcription and do not recruit co-repressors it has been shown that, like other steroid receptors, they bind to co-repressors in the presence of certain antagonists [19,24].

As mentioned above, binding of the ligand to the receptor induces a conformational change that leads to co-activator recruitment. Most of the co-activators that interact with the receptors in a ligand- and AF-2-dependent manner do so through a small signature motif called the LxxLL NR box (where x is any amino-acid) motifs that are embedded in a short α-helical peptide (see [22,23] for a review). These NR boxes are necessary and sufficient for ligand-dependent direct interaction with a cognate surface in the nuclear receptor ligand-binding domain that constitutes the transcriptional activation function AF-2. This surface corresponds to a hydrophobic cleft with 'charge clamps', to which helix H12 contributes when repositioned on the surface of the ligand-binding domain upon ligand binding. This hydrophobic cleft accommodates the amphipathic LxxLL NR box helix of co-activators as has been revealed by X-ray crystallography (reviewed in [6] and [19]).

Most nuclear receptors, such as ERs require a large variety of co-activator proteins for their transcriptional activation activities [23,25]. Such co-activators, are now known to act in three major complexes: (*i*) the ATP-dependent chromatin remodelling SWI/SNF/BRG complexes which contain nuclear ATPases such as BRG-1 or BRM that are closely related to the yeast Swi-2 protein; (*ii*) the p160 multiprotein complex which possesses intrinsic histone acetyltransferase activity. This multiprotein complex includes histone acetyltransferases (the p160 family co-activators SRC-1/NCoA-1, TIF2/GRIP1/NCoA-2, and pCIP/ACTR/AIB1/RAC3/NCoA-3), the p300 and CBP transcriptional integrators, and the CBP/p300-associated factor (pCAF) as well as

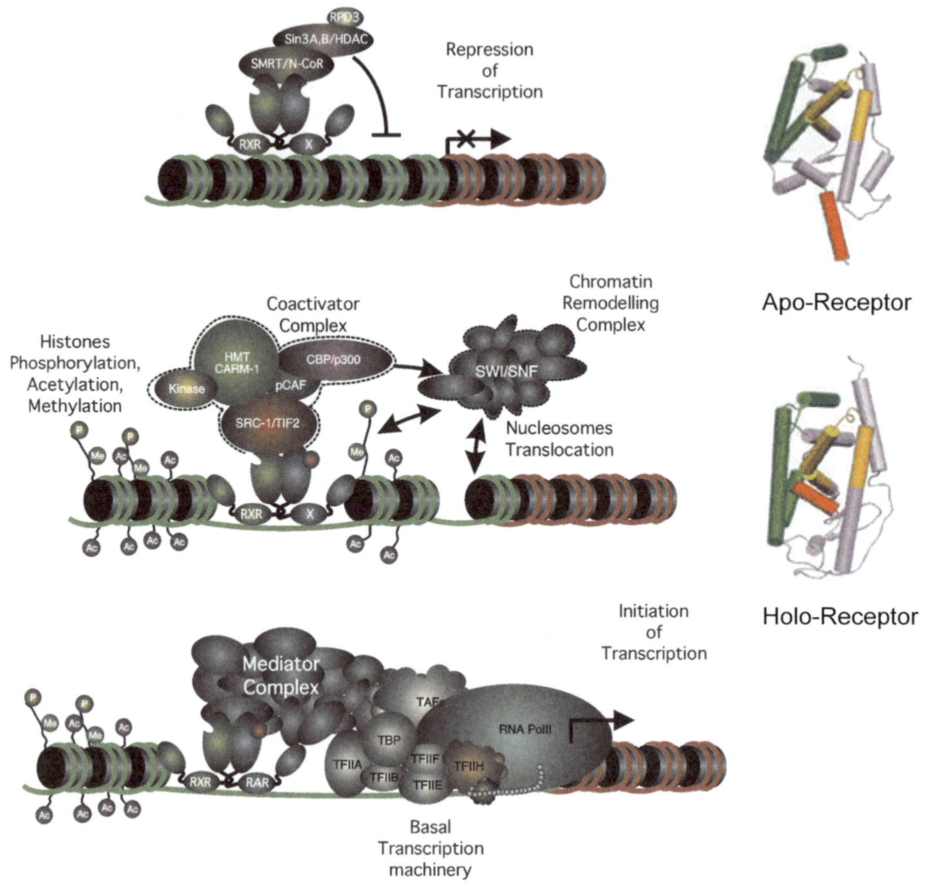

Figure 2. An oversimplified model of NR mode of action. In the absence of ligand most NRs in the apo form (right) are bound to DNA as dimers and actively repress target genes through the recruitment of co-repressor complexes that induce histone deacetylation. The ligand promotes a conformational change (holo form, right) that led to the release of co-repressors and the binding of co-activators that mediate histone acetylation and gene activation. In a second step the mediator complex leading to transcriptional initiation replaces co-activators.

numerous other proteins such as the protein-methyltransferase CARM1, the RNA co-activator SRA, or the helicases p68 and p72; (*iii*) the mediator-like protein complexes that is called DRIP, TRAP, ARC, SMCC or PBP complex which among others contain the DRIP205/TRAP220 protein that interact with ligand-activated nuclear receptors in an AF-2-dependent manner (see Figure 2 as well as [4] and [23] for reviews).

A sequential model of NR-mediated transcriptional initiation suggests that the p160 proteins dissociate, subsequent to their acetylation that decreases their ability to interact with the receptors, or their degradation by the proteasome. This initial chromatin-modifying step carried out by p160 co-activators has to be followed by the actual recruitment of the RNA polymerase II holoenzyme. Activated NRs can recruit the transcriptional machinery through their association with members of the mammalian mediator (TRAP/DRIP complex), which directly contacts components of the basal transcription machinery (see [4,19,22,23,25] and references therein).

All these entities are composed of several subunits that are associated through protein-protein interactions. The precise composition and activity of these complexes is variable from one tissue or one promoter to another and these complexes can be modified at distinct steps of the transcription initiation process but the molecular details of these processes are still far from being clear. Of course other co-activators that are not directly linked to these three major complexes exist (see [22]). Indeed, there are a number of additional proteins that have been proposed as NR co-activators based on simple criteria of ligand-dependent binding to NRs and/or ability to synergize NR-mediated transactivation evaluated by transfection-based assays (see [23] and references therein). The question whether these additional molecules play a totally independent role or are linked to the three complex types is still under intense scrutiny in a number of laboratories as is the question of the relationship between all these proteins and the basic transcription machinery, including TBP-associated factors (TAFs).

3. NR Ligands: A Complex and Evolving Notion

As discussed above, the ligand-binding pocket is an important structural feature of NRs, at least for the liganded receptors, since the first step of receptor activation is initiated by ligand binding. It is generally located behind helix 3 and in the front of helices 7 and 10, and is lined with hydrophobic amino-acids. Few polar residues at the deep end of the pocket near the β-turn act as anchoring points for the cognate ligand or play an essential role in its correct positioning, thus reinforcing the selectivity of the pocket. The specificity of ligand binding is also determined by the shape of the pocket, which can vary greatly from one receptor to another.

NRs were first described as high-affinity hormone receptors (Kd at the nanomolar range) highly selective for the binding of well-characterized hormones. Estrogen receptors, glucocorticoid receptors and thyroid hormone receptors are classical examples of such receptors. The thyroid hormone receptor, for example, binds T3 as a high-affinity physiological ligand and the affinity for T4, the precursor of T3 is 10-fold lower [26]. Similarly, reverse T3, which like T3 contains 3 iodines but placed in different positions, has a much lower affinity, exemplifying the very strong selectivity of the receptor. Given the importance of these molecules in human physiology, NR genes were considered as major targets to identify new hormones behaving in a similar way and numerous large screens to find similar high-affinity selective ligands for orphan receptors were initiated (see Figure 3).

It rapidly became clear that the situation was much more complex and plastic. The fact that retinoic acid, which is not a hormone but rather a morphogen or a growth factor was a high-affinity ligand for a nuclear receptor was a first indication that the ligands for NRs were much more diverse than expected. Then, ligands derived from food and/or intermediate cholesterol and fatty acid metabolism were identified for receptors such as PPARs, LXRs or FXRs. The fact that it was the case of the PPARs that provided the first hints in this new direction is interesting to mention. In fact PPARs (hence their bizarre name) were first discovered as high-affinity receptors for molecules known to promote peroxisome proliferation and hepatocarcinogenesis in rodents [27]. It became then clear that the transcriptional activity of the PPARs was also regulated in transfection assays by fatty acids but these molecules were considered as activators and not as *bona fide* ligands. This distinction is important: an activator can promote the transcriptional activity of a NR without being a real ligand since it can be the precursor of this ligand [1]. At the same time PPARs were shown to bind fibrates that were already known as potent hypolipidemic drugs that were used in the clinic. We now believe that there is a multitude of PPAR ligands and that these ligands are different in the three PPAR genes (PPARα, β and γ) and even

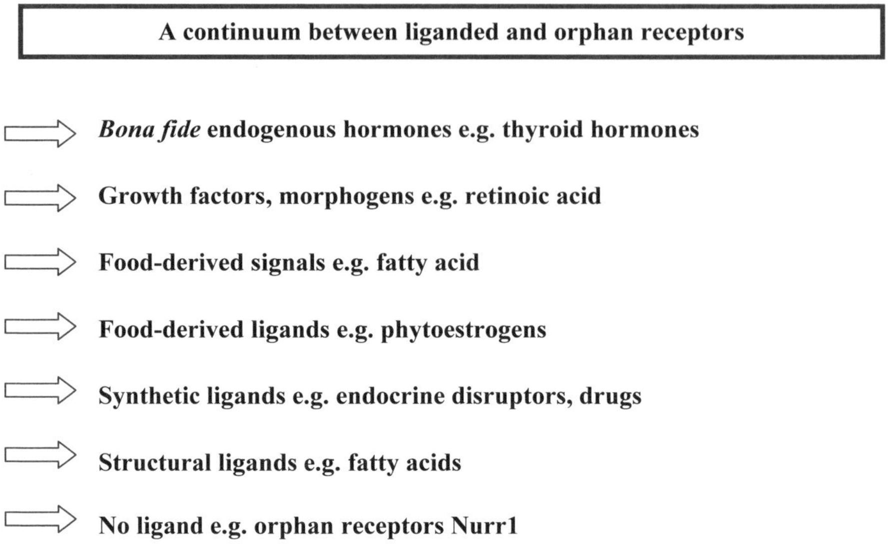

A continuum between liganded and orphan receptors

⟹   ***Bona fide*** **endogenous hormones e.g. thyroid hormones**

⟹   **Growth factors, morphogens e.g. retinoic acid**

⟹   **Food-derived signals e.g. fatty acid**

⟹   **Food-derived ligands e.g. phytoestrogens**

⟹   **Synthetic ligands e.g. endocrine disruptors, drugs**

⟹   **Structural ligands e.g. fatty acids**

⟹   **No ligand e.g. orphan receptors Nurr1**

Figure 3. A schematic illustration of the various mode of interaction between small hydrophobic molecules and nuclear receptors.

between different species. Interestingly, the endogenous ligands for PPARs are still a matter of investigation because many researchers in the field are still convinced that a "real" *bona fide* ligand with high-affinity and selectivity exists for these receptors. Nevertheless, given the prevalent view today suggesting that PPARs act as lipid sensors that translate changes in lipid/fatty acid levels from the diet into metabolic activity leading to lipid storage or fatty acid catabolism, it is likely that a multitude of ligands exist [28]. The situation is striking in that at the same time a large number of synthetic compounds can behave as PPAR ligands with high-affinity (nanomolar range) and selectivity. Thiazolidinediones such as pioglitazone or rosiglitazone or fibrates such as fenofibrates are well-known agonists of PPARγ and PPARα respectively used for treatment of diabetes and dyslipidemia. This example, which parallels very closely what has been found later on for LXR (recently described as a glucose sensor [29]) or FXR exemplifies how the field has conceptually moved from specific ligands for receptors such as TRs to regulators of the activity of metabolic sensors such as PPARs [30].

The estrogen receptor is in fact an interesting case to mention in this discussion because it provides a link between the "receptors" and the "sensors". ERs are clearly receptors of 17β-estradiol, the natural estrogen present in human. Nevertheless the diversity of molecules that can bind to estrogen receptors is enormous since ERα and ERβ are the targets of many pollutants and man-made chemicals, collectively referred to as endocrine disruptors, that are known to affect the reproductive physiology of humans and animals [3,31]. Bisphenol A, the insecticide DDT, alkyl phenols or phthalates are examples of such compounds [31]. Even more interestingly, plant-derived compounds such as genistein (found in soy); flavonoids such as luteolin (found in alfalfa) are classical examples of these types of molecules called phytoestrogens [31]. The ERs are thus able to sense the level of these compounds present in the food and to precisely regulate the transcriptional activity of the organisms in response to these compounds. Whether this represents an ancestral system from which high-affinity estrogens binding as then be elaborated is still an open, and active, question. Interestingly VDR, that is a receptor for vitamin D (1,25(OH)2D3) but also for bile acids such as lithocholic acid, provides another example of a high-affinity receptor whose selectivity is finally wider than expected [32].

The xenobiotic sensors PXR and CAR are also interesting to mention on the road to a more and more diverse relationship between NRs and small molecules (reviewed in [30]). Both receptors are known to bind to an amazingly large number of compounds. They respond to a wide variety of toxic foreign compounds (hyperforin, rifampicin, TCBOBOP etc.) but also to potentially toxic endogenous compounds called endobiotics (e.g. bile acids, oxysterol precursors etc.). CAR was even described as a receptor that can be de-activated by its ligand (androgen metabolites androstanol and androstenol), that are thus behaving as inverse agonists [33]. Interestingly the 3D-structure of the ligand-binding domain of human PXR complexed with the cholesterol-lowering drug SR12813 reveals that the very large ligand-binding cavity contains a small number of polar residues, permitting SR12813 to bind in three distinct orientations [34]. Thus a unique ligand can find its place in a pocket in three different orientations, clearly highlighting the versatility of this receptor.

At this stage it is important to mention a series of bizarre observations that considerably broaden the list of possible behaviours in the ligand-receptor relationships. First two molecules of a PPARγ ligand, FMOC-L-Leucine, have been shown to bind simultaneously to the large pocket of the receptor [35]. Interestingly, a second ligand-binding site has been recently shown to exist in the case of ERβ. Indeed a well-known ligand, the estrogen antagonist 4-hydroxytamoxifen (HT) can occupy not only the core binding pocket within the ligand-binding domain of ERβ but also a second site on its surface that overlaps with the hydrophobic groove of the co-activator recognition surface [36]. These striking observations have to be confirmed and extended before their potential in terms of drug design can be assessed but this clearly shows that even on well-known receptors or ligands new and amazing observations are still possible. Recently it was discovered that the drosophila receptor E75 contains a heme prosthetic group, and the oxidation state of this heme, modified through the binding of either nitric oxide or carbon monoxide molecules, determines whether the receptor can interact with its partner DHR3 [37]. Whether this is also true for the vertebrate orthologue of E75, the orphan receptors Rev-erbs, and its partner DHR3 (the orphan receptors RORs) is still unknown.

The example of E75 allows us to describe orphan receptors (reviewed in [38]). If some orphan receptors such Nurr1 are considered as «real» orphans since the crystal structure of their LBD does not reveal any pocket, some others are clearly ligand-regulated [39]. This is the case of ERRs for which several activators are described but are still considered as orphan receptors because they have no endogenous ligand [40]. This may also be the case for SF-1 or LRH-1 that are somehow on the path to becoming adopted orphans since their transcriptional activity can be regulated by phosphatidyl inositol [41]. Several cases of orphan receptors (HNF4, USP) permanently associated with fortuitous ligands that were captured in the ligand-binding pocket during over-expression in bacteria should nevertheless be taken as cautionary tales before claiming that a new ligand has been identified (see [38] for a review).

These examples clearly show that the notion of NR ligand should be revisited since the view that a ligand is a high-affinity and specific molecule that binds to a receptor is not describing correctly the complex reality. The case of RXR which was described as a *bona fide* receptor for 9-*cis* retinoic acid, a compound that is not found in significant amount *in vivo* and was later shown to behave as a lipid sensor, exemplifies how a more modern definition of a NR ligand would be important [42]. It is clear that three characteristics that should be present for a molecule to be defined as a NR ligand are: a) the possibility to be exchanged (that is to freely enter and leave the pocket), b) the presence *in vivo* at relevant concentrations and c) the ability to promote a conformational change of the LBD [4,19].

4. SNuRMs

Many studies have explored the structural and functional basis of ligand selectivity and the interested reader should start by looking the following reviews [6,14,19] for an overview of this rapidly evolving field. As discussed above, the activity of NRs is mediated by the LBD helix H12, the position of which depends on whether ligand is bound, and determines the ability of the receptor to recruit co-factors. Binding of an agonist triggers a mechanism by which H12 is stabilized in the so-called active conformation, thereby creating a surface of interaction with short LxxLL motifs of co-activators. Conversely, binding of an antagonist keeps helix H12 out of the active position. In the absence of ligand or in the presence of certain antagonists, co-repressors can bind to NRs through a longer LxxxI/HxxxL/I helical motif to the same surface as the co-activators with H12 displaced from the active orientation. This general concept of a molecular switch involved in the activation and inhibition of receptors mostly derives from X-ray crystallography experiments and does not fully explain the functional behaviour of ligands such as partial agonists, antagonists or inverse agonists [19]. This is mainly due to the fact that the regulation of the transcriptional activity of NRs is a highly dynamic process, a feature that is often not well illustrated by static crystal structures. An important point to realise is that the ligand-binding pocket is a highly adaptative structure that can adapt to various ligand shapes. Thus different ligands can induce slightly different conformations of helix 12, thereby generating different surfaces of the receptors that thus allow the recruitment of different types of co-activator complexes. The fact that a large number of such co-activators exist and that a wide variety of ligand-induced conformations of the LBD have been described, shows that there is an enormous amount of variation that can be explored for drug design. This adaptability of the ligand-binding pocket is at the basis of the effects of Selective Nuclear Receptor Modulators (SNuRMs) that are nuclear receptor ligands having cell or tissue-specific activities [4,19]. In fact, SNuRMs can simply be viewed as partial agonists-antagonists. Ligands with such characteristics have been developed for a number of NRs, such as ERs (SERM), AR (SARM), and PPARs (SPPARM) [43]. Their mixed agonistic/antagonistic properties are associated with differential recruitment of co-activators versus co-repressors and the tissue-selective expression profiles of these co-regulators explain the tissue-selective effect of the ligand [43-45].

As often in the past, it was the study of estrogen receptors, whose pleiotropy in terms of ligand recognition has been illustrated above, that has provided the first conceptual and functional examples along these lines. The "historical" SERMs such as raloxifene and tamoxifen whose therapeutic effect depends on their anti-estrogenic activities are prototypical examples [46,47]. In contrast to its effect in breast cancer cells in which it is anti-estrogenic, in the uterus, tamoxifen is estrogenic. In fact both tamoxifen and raloxifene induce the recruitment of co-repressors to target gene promoters in mammary cells. In cells of the uterine endometrium, however, tamoxifen, but not raloxifene, acts like estrogen by stimulating the recruitment of co-activators to a subset of target genes. The estrogen-like activity of tamoxifen in the uterus requires a high level of a specific co-activator SRC-1 that is effectively more expressed in uterus than in mammary gland. Thus cell-type- and promoter-specific differences in co-regulator recruitment determine the cellular response to SERMs. Indeed over-expression of SRC-1 or of the co-repressors NCoR and SMRT enhances or represses the partial agonist activity of tamoxifen, respectively. As a result, the overall balance and relative concentrations of co-activators and co-repressors can determine the estrogenic activity of tamoxifen. Therefore, cell-type and promoter-specific differences in co-regulator recruitment determine the cellular response to SNuRMs [19,43].

Originally defined on the estrogen receptor, the SNuRMs concept is now believed to be true for most if not all nuclear receptors and is thus extremely promising in terms of drug design since its application should allow defining drugs with much less severe adverse effects [4]. Ideally it may even be possible, by applying systematically genome-wide transcriptional studies to define active molecules that will precisely turn on or off a given subset of target genes. New technologies such as chromatin immunoprecipitation, coupled with DNA chips will certainly allow defining more precisely the concept of NR target gene [48-50]. There is no doubt that exciting discoveries, both at the level of basic and clinical endocrinology, will come from these new approaches.

Acknowledgement

Given the extreme dynamism of this field, I would like to apologize for all colleagues whose work could not be cited due to space limitations. I thank G. Benoit and M. Theodosiou for critical reading of this paper. The work from my laboratory is supported by CNRS, MENRT, ARC, ANR and Region Rhone-Alpes.

References

[1]   V. Laudet and H. Gronemeyer. The Nuclear Receptor FactsBook, Academic Press (2002).

[2]   J. Matthews and J.A. Gustafsson. Estrogen signaling: a subtle balance between ER alpha and ER beta. *Mol. Interv.* **3** (2003) 281-292.

[3]   D. Crews and J.A. McLachlan. Epigenetics, evolution, endocrine disruption, health, and disease. *Endocrinology* **147** (2006) S4-10.

[4]   H. Gronemeyer, J.A. Gustafsson, V. Laudet. Principles for modulation of the nuclear receptor superfamily. *Nat. Rev. Drug Discov.* **3** (2004) 950-964.

[5]   D.M. Lonard and C.L. Smith. Molecular perspectives on selective estrogen receptor modulators (SERMs): progress in understanding their tissue-specific agonist and antagonist actions. *Steroids* **67** (2002) 15-24.

[6]   G. Benoit, M. Malewicz, T. Perlmann. Digging deep into the pockets of orphan nuclear receptors: insights from structural studies. *Trends Cell Biol.* **14** (2004) 369-376.

[7]   H. Escriva, R. Safi, C. Hanni *et al.* Ligand binding was acquired during evolution of nuclear receptors. *Proc. Natl. Acad. Sci. U.S.A.* **94** (1997) 6803-6808.

[8]   C. Phelps, V. Gburcik, E. Suslova *et al.* Fungi and animals may share a common ancestor to nuclear receptors. *Proc. Natl. Acad. Sci. U.S.A.* **103** (2006) 7077-7081.

[9]   H. Escriva Garcia, V. Laudet, M. Robinson-Rechavi. Nuclear receptors are markers of animal genome evolution. *J. Struct. Funct. Genomics* **3** (2003) 177-184.

[10] H. Escriva, S. Bertrand, V. Laudet. The evolution of the nuclear receptor superfamily. *Essays Biochem.* **40** (2004) 11-26.

[11] W. Wu, E.G. Niles, H. Hirai *et al.* Evolution of a novel subfamily of nuclear receptors with members that each contain two DNA binding domains. *BMC Evol. Biol.* **7** (2007) 27.

[12] J.W. Thornton, E. Need, D. Crews. Resurrecting the ancestral steroid receptor: ancient origin of estrogen signaling. *Science* **301** (2003) 1714-1717.

[13] Nuclear Receptors Nomenclature Committee. A unified nomenclature system for the nuclear receptor superfamily. *Cell* **97** (1999) 161-163.

[14] A.C. Steinmetz, J.P. Renaud, D. Moras. Binding of ligands and activation of transcription by nuclear receptors. *Annu. Rev. Biophys. Biomol. Struct.* **30** (2001) 329-359.

[15] K. De Bosscher, W. Vanden Berghe, G. Haegeman. The interplay between the glucocorticoid receptor and nuclear factor-kappaB or activator protein-1: molecular mechanisms for gene repression. *Endocr. Rev.* **24** (2003) 488-522.

[16] J.S. Carroll and M. Brown. Estrogen receptor target gene: an evolving concept. *Mol. Endocrinol.* **20** (2006) 1707-1714.

[17] J.F. Couse and K.S. Korach. Estrogen receptor null mice: what have we learned and where will they lead us? *Endocr. Rev.* **20** (1999) 358-417. Erratum in: *Endocr. Rev.* **20** (1999) 459.

[18] K.F. Koehler, L.A. Helguero, L.A. Haldosen *et al.* Reflections on the discovery and significance of estrogen receptor beta. *Endocr. Rev.* **26** (2005) 465-478.

[19] P. Germain, B. Staels, C. Dacquet *et al.* Overview of nomenclature of nuclear receptors. *Pharmacol. Rev.* **58** (2006) 685-704.

[20] W. Bourguet, M. Ruff, P. Chambon *et al.* Crystal structure of the ligand-binding domain of the human nuclear receptor RXR-alpha. *Nature* **375** (1995) 377-382. Comment in: *Nature* **375** (1995) 359-360.

[21]   J.M. Wurtz, W. Bourguet, J.P. Renaud *et al.* A canonical structure for the ligand-binding domain of nuclear receptors. *Nat. Struct. Biol.* **3** (1996) 87-94. Erratum in: *Nat. Struct. Biol.* **3** (1996) 206. Comment in: *Nat. Struct. Biol.* **3** (1996) 113-115.

[22]   N.J. McKenna, R.B. Lanz, B.W. O'Malley. Nuclear receptor coregulators: cellular and molecular biology. *Endocr. Rev.* **20** (1999) 321-344.

[23]   M.G. Rosenfeld, V.V. Lunyak, C.K. Glass. Sensors and signals: a coactivator/corepressor/epigenetic code for integrating signal-dependent programs of transcriptional response. *Genes Dev.* **20** (2006) 1405-1428.

[24]   K. Dahlman-Wright, V. Cavailles, S.A. Fuqua *et al.* International Union of Pharmacology. LXIV. Estrogen receptors. *Pharmacol. Rev.* **58** (2006) 773-781.

[25]   L.P. Freedman. Increasing the complexity of coactivation in nuclear receptor signaling. *Cell* **97** (1999) 5-8.

[26]   F. Flamant, J.D. Baxter, D. Forrest *et al.* International Union of Pharmacology. LIX. The pharmacology and classification of the nuclear receptor superfamily: thyroid hormone receptors. *Pharmacol. Rev.* **58** (2006) 705-711.

[27]   L. Michalik, J. Auwerx, J.P. Berger *et al.* International Union of Pharmacology. LXI. Peroxisome proliferator-activated receptors. *Pharmacol. Rev.* **58** (2006) 726-741.

[28]   A.K. Hihi, L. Michalik, W. Wahli. PPARs: transcriptional effectors of fatty acids and their derivatives. *Cell. Mol. Life Sci.* **59** (2002) 790-798.

[29]   N. Mitro, P.A. Mak, L. Vargas *et al.* The nuclear receptor LXR is a glucose sensor. *Nature* **445** (2007) 219-223.

[30]   D.D. Moore, S. Kato, W. Xie *et al.* International Union of Pharmacology. LXII. The NR1H and NR1I receptors: constitutive androstane receptor, pregnene X receptor, farnesoid X receptor alpha, farnesoid X receptor beta, liver X receptor alpha, liver X receptor beta, and vitamin D receptor. *Pharmacol. Rev.* **58** (2006) 742-759.

[31]   J.A. McLachlan. Environmental signaling: what embryos and evolution teach us about endocrine disrupting chemicals. *Endocr. Rev.* **22** (2001) 319-341.

[32]   M. Makishima, T.T. Lu, W. Xie *et al.* Vitamin D receptor as an intestinal bile acid sensor. *Science* **296** (2002) 1313-1316.

[33]   B.M. Forman, I. Tzameli, H.S. Choi *et al.* Androstane metabolites bind to and deactivate the nuclear receptor CAR-beta. *Nature* **395** (1998) 612-615. Comment in: *Nature* **395** (1998) 543-544.

[34]   R.E. Watkins, G.B. Wisely, L.B. Moore *et al.* The human nuclear xenobiotic receptor PXR: structural determinants of directed promiscuity. *Science* **292** (2001) 2329-2333.

[35]   S. Rocchi, F. Picard, J. Vamecq *et al.* A unique PPARgamma ligand with potent insulin-sensitizing yet weak adipogenic activity. *Mol. Cell* **8** (2001) 737-747.

[36]   Y. Wang, N.Y. Chirgadze, S.L. Briggs *et al.* A second binding site for hydroxytamoxifen within the coactivator-binding groove of estrogen receptor beta. *Proc. Natl. Acad. Sci. U.S.A.* **103** (2006) 9908-9911.

[37]   J. Reinking, M.M. Lam, K. Pardee *et al.* The Drosophila nuclear receptor e75 contains heme and is gas responsive. *Cell* **122** (2005) 195-207. Comment in: *Cell* **122** (2005) 151-153.

[38]   G. Benoit, A. Cooney, V. Giguère *et al.* International Union of Pharmacology. LXVI. Orphan nuclear receptors. *Pharmacol. Rev.* **58** (2006) 798-836

[39]   Z. Wang, G. Benoit, J. Liu *et al.* Structure and function of Nurr1 identifies a class of ligand-independent nuclear receptors. *Nature* **423** (2003) 555-560.

[40]   B. Horard and J.M. Vanacker. Estrogen receptor-related receptors: orphan receptors desperately seeking a ligand. *J. Mol. Endocrinol.* **31** (2003) 349-357.

[41]   I.N. Krylova, E.P. Sablin, J. Moore *et al.* Structural analyses reveal phosphatidyl inositols as ligands for the NR5 orphan receptors SF-1 and LRH-1. *Cell* **120** (2005) 343-355. Comment in: *Cell Metab.* **1** (2005) 153-155.

[42]   P. Germain, P. Chambon, G. Eichele *et al.* International Union of Pharmacology. LXIII. Retinoid X receptors. *Pharmacol. Rev.* **58** (2006) 760-772.

[43]   C.L. Smith, B.W. O'Malley. Coregulator function: a key to understanding tissue specificity of selective receptor modulators. *Endocr. Rev.* **25** (2004) 45-71.

[44]   Z. Liu, D. Auboeuf, J. Wong *et al.* Coactivator/corepressor ratios modulate PR-mediated transcription by the selective receptor modulator RU486. *Proc. Natl. Acad. Sci. U.S.A.* **99** (2002) 7940-7944.

[45]   P. Webb, P. Nguyen, P.J. Kushner. Differential SERM effects on corepressor binding dictate ERalpha activity in vivo. *J. Biol. Chem.* **278** (2003) 6912-6920.

[46]   Y. Shang, X. Hu, J. DiRenzo *et al.* Cofactor dynamics and sufficiency in estrogen receptor-regulated transcription. *Cell* **103** (2000) 843-852.

[47]   Y. Shang and M. Brown. Molecular determinants for the tissue specificity of SERMs. *Science* **295** (2002) 2465-2468. Comment in: *Science* **295** (2002) 2380-2381.

[48]　R. Metivier, G. Reid, F. Gannon. Transcription in four dimensions: nuclear receptor-directed initiation of gene expression. *EMBO Rep.* **7** (2006) 161-167.

[49]　J.S. Carroll, X.S. Liu, A.S. Brodsky *et al.* Chromosome-wide mapping of estrogen receptor binding reveals long-range regulation requiring the forkhead protein FoxA1. *Cell* **122** (2005) 33-43.

[50]　C.Y. Lin, A. Strom, V.B. Vega *et al.* Discovery of estrogen receptor alpha target genes and response elements in breast tumor cells. *Genome Biol.* **5** (2004) R66.

Metabolic Control by LXR

Jean Louis Junien

*Laboratoires Fournier, a Solvay Pharmaceuticals company, 50 rue de Dijon, 21121 Daix,
France*

Abstract. Atherosclerotic coronary artery disease is still the leading cause of
mortality in industrialised countries. This is largely related to the current tremendous
increase of the prevalence of obesity, metabolic syndrome and diabetes. Therefore
new strategies have to be developed for stopping such an epidemic situation. Drugs
acting through the nuclear receptor LXR may offer an additional benefit or an
alternative approach to current therapies since LXR receptors modulate not only the
genes controlling the Reverse Cholesterol Transport (RCT) but also genes involved
in pathways which are altered in metabolic diseases.

Originally identified as orphan members of the nuclear receptor
superfamily, Liver X Receptors exist as two isoforms, LXRα and LXRβ. Oxysterols
were identified as the putative physiological ligands for the LXRs, and additional
studies have demonstrated that these receptors act as sensors for these cholesterol
metabolites and are essential components of a physiological feedback loop
regulating cholesterol metabolism and transport. LXR pathway may have also an
important role in glucose metabolism since many reports now have shown that
LXR-activation can be protective in genetic diabetes models in rodent, improve
glucose tolerance and facilitate pancreas insulin secretion.

However the usefulness of LXRs as pharmacological targets has been
questioned by the effect of systemic LXR-activation on the expression of hepatic
lipogenic genes directly and via activation of hepatic sterol regulatory element-
binding protein-1C (SREBP-1C) leading to hypertriglyceridemia and hepatic
steatosis. Successful development of LXR-based therapeutics will therefore require
methods to exploit the beneficial aspects of LXR-activation whereas avoiding these
unwanted side effects.

Keywords. LXR receptors, oxysterols, Reverse Cholesterol Transport,
atherosclerosis, macrophage cholesterol efflux, ABCA transporters, SREBP-1C,
lipogenesis, diabetes

Introduction

Atherosclerotic coronary artery disease (CAD) is the leading cause of mortality in
industrialised countries. Despite the discovery in the last two decades of efficient drugs for
the treatment of the multiple cardiovascular risk factors, it is predicted that in the next two
decades CAD will become the leading cause of death worldwide. This is largely related to
the tremendous increase of the prevalence of obesity, metabolic syndrome and diabetes [1].
New therapeutic strategies have to be developed for stopping such an epidemic situation.

Many biological mechanisms are involved in the initiation, progression and
activation of atherosclerotic lesions with one of these being the uptake of oxidised low-
density lipoprotein (LDL) by macrophages present in the fatty streaks/plaques in the arterial
wall. This results in the accumulation of cholesterol esters, leading to the formation of
foam-cells. Other biological processes are triggered, including the recruitment of
inflammatory cells and production of inflammatory mediators. Subsequent activation of

atherosclerotic plaques can result in rupture of the fibrous cap, exposing the thrombogenic contents of the plaque core, leading to thrombotic clot formation, myocardial infarction or cerebral ischemia.

Drugs acting through the nuclear receptor LXR may offer an additional benefit or an alternative approach to current therapies since LXR receptors modulate not only the genes controlling the Reverse Cholesterol Transport (RCT) but also genes involved in pathways which are altered in metabolic diseases [2-5]. It is also hoped that such drug may reverse plaque progression by effluxing out cholesterol from macrophages. A first demonstration of a true reversal effect has been provided recently with the use of the ApoA1 Milano in an IVUS study [6]. Whether this could translate into a true curative clinical effect remain to be demonstrated in clinical studies in the future.

Originally identified as orphan members of the nuclear receptor superfamily, Liver X Receptors exist as two isoforms, LXRα and LXRβ. The two isoforms display distinct patterns of expression with LXRα being primarily expressed in liver, intestine, and kidney, whereas LXR is expressed ubiquitously. LXRα and LXRβ heterodimerize with RXR and control transcription by binding to a direct repeat type 4 LXR response element (LXRE) located in the promoter of their target genes. Oxysterols were identified as the putative physiological ligands for the LXRs [7,8], and additional studies have demonstrated that these receptors act as sensors for these cholesterol metabolites and are essential components of a physiological feedback loop regulating cholesterol metabolism and transport [3].

More recently Mitro *et al* [9] have reported that D-glucose and D-glucose-6-phosphate also binds and stimulates the transcriptional activity of the LXRα,β receptors. According Mitro *et al* [9], glucose would activate LXR at physiological concentrations in the liver and induces expression of LXR-target genes with efficacy similar to that of oxysterols, providing an integrated relationship between hepatic glucose metabolism and fatty acid synthesis. This moreover add to the putative role of LXR in glucose metabolism itself since many reports now have shown that LXR-activation can be protective in genetic diabetes models in rodent [10], improve glucose tolerance and facilitate pancreas insulin secretion [10-11].

However the usefulness of LXRs as pharmacological targets has been questioned by the effect of systemic LXR-activation on the expression of hepatic lipogenic genes directly and via activation of hepatic sterol regulatory element-binding protein-1C (SREBP-1C) leading to hypertriglyceridemia and hepatic steatosis [12,13]. Successful development of LXR-based therapeutics will therefore require methods to exploit the beneficial aspects of LXR-activation whereas avoiding these unwanted side effects. This article reviews the different mechanisms and targets that are affected by LXR ligands and their potential therapeutic interest in the treatment of metabolic diseases and atherosclerosis.

Role of LXR Receptors in the Cholesterol Metabolism

LXR-agonists Increase Reverse Cholesterol Transport

Reverse Cholesterol Transport (RCT) is the process by which cholesterol is transported from peripheral tissues and becomes incorporated in high-density lipoproteins (HDL) which are transported to the liver for metabolism. Cholesterol and biliary salts may be then either reabsorbed in the intestine or excreted in the feces. Epidemiological studies and clinical trials have identified that decreased levels of HDL (and elevated levels of LDL) are pro-atherogenic [14]. The ATP-binding cassette transporter A1 (ABCA1) is a crucial component in the process of RCT and has been shown to be modulated by the Liver X Receptors [12-15]. Activation of LXR in macrophages induces ABCA1 expression and stimulates ApoA-I–mediated cholesterol efflux [8]. Consistent with their ability to activate the reverse cholesterol transport, LXR ligands increase high-density lipoprotein cholesterol in mice. Patients with Tangiers disease, and the milder heterozygous form, familial hypoalphalipoproteinemia (FHA), have been shown to possess mutations in the ABCA1 gene. In Tangiers disease this homozygous mutation results in a virtual absence of circulating HDL cholesterol, and a premature onset of atherosclerosis [15-18]. Therefore, increasing RCT through modulation of the ABCA1 pathway represents an attractive potential therapeutic mechanism for the treatment of atherosclerosis. ABCG1, another member of the ABC transporter family, is also strongly induced by cholesterol loading of macrophages and was recently identified as a direct target of LXRs in mouse and human cells. Induction of ABCG1 may provide an additional pathway for cholesterol efflux from macrophages or may act in concert with ABCA1 [19].

Another mechanism that may contribute to the effect of LXR-activation on reverse cholesterol transport is the induction of ApoE gene expression in macrophages [20]. It is moreover well established that ApoE has a protective role in atherogenesis. Loss of macrophage ApoE leads to increased lesions, whereas over-expression of ApoE in these cells is protective [21]. The ApoC gene cluster (ApoC-I, ApoC-II, and ApoC-IV) is also induced by LXRs in macrophages [22].

Indeed Naik *et al* [23] have reported in mice that administration of a synthetic LXR-agonist increases the reverse transport of cholesterol from macrophages to feces *in vivo*. They showed that mice treated with the synthetic LXR-agonist GW3965 have significantly higher macrophage-derived 3H-cholesterol in plasma and feces over 48 hours than vehicle-treated in 3 different mouse models, including wild-type mice and knock-out mice models of atherosclerosis. LXR has been reported to increase CETP expression in human and primate cells but mice are lacking the CETP gene. Naik *et al* [23] also studied the effect of GW3965 on macrophage RCT in *ApoB*/CETP double transgenic mice, which exhibit a human-like lipoprotein distribution. Treatment of the *ApoB*/CETP double transgenic mice with GW3965 resulted in a significant increase in macrophage RCT, suggesting that an LXR-agonist promotes the rate of macrophage RCT *in vivo* even in the presence of CETP expression. However, the magnitude of the increase in macrophage RCT with GW3965 was less than that seen in wild-type.

Recent data [24] suggest that the intestine may play a role in directly excreting plasma-derived cholesterol into the feces, thus serving as a liver-independent pathway for RCT. Indeed, an LXR-agonist was shown to increase fecal excretion of neutral sterols independent of biliary sterol secretion. In this paradigm, treatment with GW3965, by up-regulating intestinal expression of genes such as ABCG5/G8, promoted direct intestinal transport of HDL 3H-cholesterol into the lumen, thus contributing to the overall increase in fecal 3H-sterol excretion and macrophage RCT.

Bruhnam *et al* [24] have shown that intestinal-specific deficiency of ABCA1 in mice results in a 30% reduction in plasma HDL cholesterol, indicating that intestinal ABCA1, in addition to hepatic ABCA1, is crucial for the maintenance of plasma HDL cholesterol levels. The LXR-agonist GW3965 significantly raised plasma HDL cholesterol levels in wild-type mice and mice lacking hepatic ABCA1, and this effect was completely abrogated in mice lacking intestinal ABCA1, thereby providing proof-of-principle that activation of intestinal ABCA1 can lead to an increase in HDL levels. This indicates that it may be possible to design LXR-agonists that activate specific genes in a tissue-specific manner.

LXR-agonists Can Protect from Atherosclerosis

Several studies have been reported which indicate that LXR and ABC1 gene may be protective in atherosclerosis. To assess the role of ABCA1 in atherosclerosis, Van Eck *et al* [25] engrafted LDLr[-/-] mice with bone marrow cells from ABCA1 deficient mice or from wild-type littermates. Absence of ABCA1 from leukocytes in treated mice leads to 60% increase in atherosclerotic lesion area. In two other studies, over-expression of ABCA1 gene was protective. Singaraja *et al* [26] crossed transgenic ApoE[-/-] mice with transgenic BAC mice who over express human ABCA1 gene (hABCA1-Tg mice). A marked decrease in the atherosclerotic lesion area was observed in the double transgenic mice compared to ApoE[-/-] littermates. In another study, Van Eck *et al* [27] transplanted bone marrow from Tg BAC mice to LDLr[-/-] mice. After 12 and 15 weeks of Western diet mean atherosclerosis area was respectively 3 and 2 times smaller compared with control transplanted mice. Selective loss of macrophage LXR-activity increased atherosclerotic lesion development, suggesting that LXR functions as endogenous inhibitor of atherogenesis [5]. Anti-atherosclerotic effects of LXR-agonists were demonstrated in murine models of atherogenesis, as the ApoE and the LDL receptor knock-out models [28,29]. LDLr[-/-] mice fed with a high-fat diet received T0901317; 3 and 10 mg/kg, during 8 weeks. No influence on plasma cholesterol was reported but a drastic triglycerides increase occurred during the first weeks of treatment, while the development of atherosclerosis was inhibited by 57-71% in comparison with control group. More interestingly, Levin *et al* [30] have reported a reversal of the plaque formation in LDL[-/-] mice fed with Western diet. The animals received Western diet for 8 weeks (baseline atherosclerosis group) and then were fed for 6 weeks more while they were administered with vehicle or T0901317 daily at 10 mg/kg. In comparison to vehicle-treated controls treatment resulted in a 70% reduction of lesion area.

Interestingly as in the macrophage, only LXRα protein was detected in the nucleus of mononuclear cells and foam-cells of human plaque lesions by Watanabe *et al* [31].

LXR-agonists Decrease Inflammatory Process

A large number of studies have shown that inflammation within the arterial wall is a risk factor for cardiovascular disease and promotes atherogenesis [32]. Besides to inducing genes involved in reverse cholesterol transport, LXRs repress *in vitro* also inflammatory genes after bacterial stimulation LXR would inhibit NFκB activation on promoters of target genes such as iNOS and IL-6. These effects are reproduced *ex vivo* in macrophages derived from wild-type, LXRα[-/-], and LXRβ[-/-] mice but not in macrophages from LXRαβ[-/-] mice, indicating that both LXR isoforms possess anti-inflammatory activity. Treatment of murine peritoneal macrophages with the synthetic LXR-agonists GW3965 or T0 901317 reduces MMP9 mRNA expression through antagonism of the NFκB signalling pathway and blunts its induction by pro-inflammatory stimuli including lipopolysaccharide, TNFα, IL-10. This effect is not observed in macrophages obtained from LXRαβ null mice [33].

Fowler *et al* [34] even showed that Liver X Receptor activators display anti-inflammatory activity in irritant and allergic contact dermatitis models, Liver X Receptor-specific inhibition of inflammation and primary cytokine production which raise the question of potential use of LXR-agonists for general inflammatory states.

LXRα and LXRβ receptors are present in human CD4-positive T-cells and activation of LXRs by the synthetic agonist T0901317 reduces Th1 expression of cytokines as IFNγ, TNFα and IL-2 [35]. These data suggest that LXRs, in addition to their modulatory action on macrophage function, may exhibit direct anti-inflammatory effects in CD4-positive lymphocytes, potentially contributing to the beneficial effects of LXR-agonist on lesion development in animal models of arteriosclerosis. The reduction in IFNγ expression is caused by an inhibition of IFNγ promoter activity. IFNγ has been shown to induce the expression of T-cell-specific chemokines from endothelial cells, thus facilitating the migration of T-cells into the vessel wall. IFNγ has been implicated in plaque destabilization through its capacity to induce the expression of matrix degrading MMPs. Therefore, a reduction of IFNγ release from activated T-cells may contribute to the beneficial effects of LXR-activator treatment on atherogenesis.

Besides their effects on macrophages and lymphocytes, Blaschke *et al* [36] have shown that LXRs are expressed and functional in human vascular smooth muscular cells (VSMC). LXR ligands suppress mitogen-induced VSMC proliferation and neointima formation in a model of rat carotid artery balloon injury. The mechanism by which LXR ligands inhibit VSMC proliferation and cell-cycle progression involves an inhibition of R*b* phosphorylation mediated through an inhibition of Skp2-dependent down-regulation of p27Kip1. Activation, migration, and proliferation in response to injury play not only a decisive role for development of atherosclerosis but are also the primary pathophysiologic mechanism resulting in the failure of procedures used to treat occlusive proliferative atherosclerotic diseases, such as post-angioplasty restenosis, transplant vasculopathy, and vein bypass graft failure.

Role of LXR in Glucose Metabolism

A second important metabolic role of LXR is to improve glucose tolerance through different mechanisms which are reported below.

LXR-agonists Decrease Blood Glucose in Rodents

Several studies have reported an anti-diabetic effect of LXR-agonists in animal model of diabetes. Cao *et al* [10] have reported an effect of T0901317 after a one week treatment in db/db mice and ZDF rat. The maximum efficacy in plasma glucose-lowering achieved with T0901317 was comparable with rosiglitazone. In ZDF rats, plasma glucose levels were significantly reduced while both plasma and liver triglycerides in db/db and ZDF rat studies increased. Obese insulin-resistant female Zucker (fa/fa) rats treated for 9 days with T0901317 revealed a significant improvement in glucose tolerance. The insulin sensitivity index, calculated as the product of the glucose AUC and the insulin AUC during the oral glucose tolerance test, was significantly improved in the treated group. Thus T0901317 effectively lowers glucose in diabetic rodents and may improve insulin sensitivity in insulin-resistant rodents but does not cause hypoglycemia in normal animals.

Laffitte *et al* [37] have investigated the ability of the synthetic LXR-agonist GW3965 to influence glucose tolerance in a model of diet-induced obesity and insulin resistance. C57BL/6 mice were maintained on a high-fat diet for 3 months. The obese mice were treated for 1 week with either vehicle or 20 mg/kg GW3965. Mice were fasted overnight, glucose-tolerance tests were performed, and plasma lipid levels were determined. Treatment with the LXR-agonist significantly improved glucose tolerance in obese mice. In contrast, GW3965 had a minimal effect on the normal glucose tolerance of lean C57BL/6 mice maintained on normal chow diet. Fasting glucose and insulin levels were not different between treated and untreated groups. There was also no statistically significant difference in free fatty acids or triglyceride levels.

LXR-agonists Decrease Neoglucogenesis and Increase Fat Synthesis in the Liver

Several reports have provided evidence that LXR ligands exert their anti-diabetic effects at least in part through suppression of neoglucogenesis. Cao *et al* [10] found significant reductions in mRNA levels of two key gluconeogenic enzymes, PEPCK and glucose-6-phosphatase (G6P), in liver samples from T0901317-treated db/db mice. PEPCK mRNA levels in T0901317-treated liver samples were reduced dose-dependently and well correlated with the glucose-lowering effects. They measured lactate-stimulated glucose output from liver slices derived from ZDF rats treated with either vehicle, T0901317 (10 mg/kg), or T0901317 (30 mg/kg). Compared with either control or a pair-fed group (matched to T0901317 30 mg/kg), T0901317 at 10 mg/kg inhibited lactate-stimulated glucose output by 80%, whereas the 30 mg/kg treatment resulted in virtually complete inhibition of glucose output. These results indicate that the LXR-agonist, T0901317, improves glucose homeostasis in diabetic rodents, at least in part, through down-regulation of key enzymes in the hepatic gluconeogenesis pathway. To determine whether the aforementioned alterations were the result of T0901317 acting directly on hepatocytes, they treated rat hepatoma Fao cells with either 0.2 nM insulin or 100 nM T0901317 or a combination of both for 24 h. The mRNA levels of PEPCK, G6P, pyruvate carboxylase, and fructose 1,6-bisphosphatase decreased dramatically upon either insulin or T0901317 treatment. The combination of both agents did not result in an additive effect. To confirm their observations, they treated rat hepatoma cells with either T0901317 or another structurally distinct synthetic LXR-agonist, GW3965, and measured PEPCK mRNA. Both compounds showed dose-dependent reductions of PEPCK mRNA levels with a good correlation with their respective described LXR potencies. These authors concluded that the *in vivo* regulation of hepatic gluconeogenic genes was a direct action of the LXR-agonist on the liver. LXR-activation alters liver metabolism in a similar manner to insulin, increasing lipogenesis and decreasing gluconeogenesis.

Laffitte *et al* [37] treated for 3 days C57B6 with either vehicle or 20 mg/kg of the synthetic LXR-agonist GW3965. LXR-agonist treatment altered expression of a number of genes linked to glucose metabolism. Treatment with GW3965 decreased expression of the transcriptional co-activator PGC-1, which is a key regulator of gluconeogenesis. This effect was confirmed *in vitro* with primary human hepatocytes. Consistent with the decrease in PGC-1, expression of the gluconeogenic enzymes phospho*enol*pyruvate carboxykinase (PEPCK) and glucose-6-phosphatase were also down-regulated by GW3965. In addition to these repressive effects, LXR-agonist induced expression of glucokinase mRNA. The glucokinase gene is positively regulated by insulin, and its expression is an important determinant of hepatic glucose metabolism leading to the elevation in hepatic glucose uptake. The mechanism whereby insulin alters gene expression in this tissue is through transcriptional up-regulation of SREBP-1C [38,39]. Transgenic expression of SREBP-1C in liver induces the entire program of fatty acid synthesis. Studies have also shown that adenoviral expression of SREBP-1C in liver induces expression of glucokinase and represses the expression of gluconeogenic genes such as PEPCK and glucose-6-phosphatase [40-43]. Thus, many of the effects of insulin on both lipid and glucose metabolism may be mediated by SREBP-1C. Because SREBP-1C is a direct target of LXR, it is possible that many of the effects of LXR-agonists in liver are the result of increased expression of SREBP-1C.

Insulin Increases LXRα mRNA in the Liver

Tobin *et al* [44] have shown a time- and dose-dependent increase in LXRα steady-state mRNA level after insulin stimulation of primary rat hepatocytes in culture. A maximal induction of 10-fold was obtained when hepatocytes were exposed to 400 nM insulin for 24 h. The induction is dependent on *de novo* synthesis of proteins. Stabilization studies using actinomycin D indicated that insulin stimulation increased the half-life of LXRα transcripts in cultured primary hepatocytes. This effect was confirmed *in vivo*, rats and mice injected with insulin had an increase of LXRα mRNA levels. Furthermore, deletion of both the LXRα and LXRβ genes (double knock-out) in mice markedly suppressed insulin-mediated induction of an entire class of enzymes involved in both fatty acid and cholesterol metabolism. The mechanisms by which insulin stimulates the transcriptional activity of LXR are presently unknown. This up-regulation could, at least partly, be the result of stabilization of the transcripts. LXR mRNA regulation by insulin is dependent on *de novo* synthesis of proteins. Further studies of the LXR promoter will be required to understand the mechanisms of this regulation. Tobin *et al* [45] have reported a PPARα-dependent fatty acid up-regulation of LXRα mRNA and protein [45], and PPARα has previously been shown to be phosphorylated in response to insulin, resulting in stimulation of basal as well as ligand-dependent transcriptional activity of PPARα [46]. PPARα could therefore be an upstream factor mediating the insulin effect on LXRα.

Glucose Acts as an Endogenous Activator of LXR Receptors in the Liver

Another piece of the puzzle was reported recently by Mitro *et al* [9] providing an explanation to this effect of LXR on the liver. They showed that glucose binds and stimulates the transcriptional activity of the Liver X Receptor (LXR), glucose activates LXR at physiological concentrations in the liver and induces expression of LXR-target genes with efficacy similar to that of oxysterols. Glucose and its derivatives stimulated significantly LXR-RXR activity in HepG2 cells grown in no glucose. D-glucose and D-glucose-6-phosphate were more potent on LXRβ than LXRα (mM range) and were weaker inducers than known LXR ligands. Using a scintillation proximity assay with (3H)T0901317 and/or (3H)D-glucose, Mitro *et al* [9] showed that D-glucose and D-glucose-6-phosphate are direct agonists of the LXRs that bind more than one site, and can work in combination with a synthetic ligand. The precise binding mode of glucose awaits the resolution of a crystal structure. In cells grown in the absence of glucose or in low glucose conditions, overnight treatment with either compound (1 µM GW3965 or 20mM D-glucose) stimulated expression of genes involved in fatty acid synthesis and repressed expression of gluconeogenic genes. They also stimulated genes involved in cholesterol homeostasis (ABCA1, ABCG5, ABCG8, ABCG1, CETP) that are not insulin-regulated and whose expression is not associated with glucose levels. The efficacy of known LXR ligands was potentiated with increasing glucose concentration, indicating that glucose can work together with established LXR ligands. Induction of LXR-dependent target genes by D-glucose and other ligands paralleled there co-factor recruitment capacity in a FRET assay and was blocked in cells transfected with siRNA against LXRα.

Fasted mice were administered with GW3965 or diets where the source of carbohydrate was exclusively sucrose or D-glucose. All diets were devoid of cholesterol to minimize endogenous generation of oxysterols. D-glucose and GW3965 induced similar changes in hepatic gene expression, triggering a pattern expected to limit hepatic glucose output and increase fatty acid synthesis as previously reported [10,37-39].

According to Mitro *et al* [9] LXR would function as a glucose sensor *in vivo* that responds to increasing liver glucose uptake. To examine the effect of insulin on glucose-stimulated, LXR-related hepatic gene expression, animals rendered insulin-deficient via streptozotocin injection were treated by glucose and GW3965 which were still able to induce expression of LXR-dependent genes, repress gluconeogenesis genes, and up-regulate fatty acid synthesis genes. Moreover, glucose was also able to induce up-regulation of LXR-target genes in the intestine of wild-type and streptozotocin-treated mice, confirming the role of glucose as a physiological LXR ligand in another tissue that faces significant glucose influx and in which the role of insulin is not as prominent.

Thus glucose and insulin may produce a concerted increase of lipogenic pathway by a increase activation and production of LXRα. LXR can sense surplus glucose, induce fatty acid synthesis, and prompt hepatic export of very-low-density lipoprotein (VLDL).

LXR-agonists Increase in Insulin Secretion in the Pancreas

LXR-activation may normalize plasma glucose levels in diabetic animals via insulin secretion. Efanov *et al* [11] have shown that human and rodent pancreatic islets express both LXRα and LXRβ isoforms. Non-β-cells expressed significantly higher LXRα levels. On the contrary, β-cells expressed LXRβ isoform in rodent. T0901317 promotes glucose-dependent insulin secretion and insulin biosynthesis in rat islets and insulin-secreting cells, whereas islets from LXRβ knock-out mice displayed lack of glucose-induced insulin secretion and increased lipid accumulation. LXRβ$^{-/-}$ mice are glucose intolerant and develop diabetes, when kept on a high-fat diet, due to impaired insulin secretion [47]. LXRβ plays an important role in controlling expression of genes crucial for the β-cell phenotype. Activation of SREBP-1, the target gene of LXRβ in β-cells, is likely the mechanism for the induction of insulin secretion [48] as well as pancreatic duodenal homeobox 1 (PDX-1) mRNA levels. PDX-1 is required for pancreas development and is critical for maintaining the differentiated β-cell phenotype. PDX-1 is a major transactivator of the insulin gene and mediates glucose-induced up-regulation of insulin expression. Induction of PDX-1 expression by SREBP-1 may be a way to increase insulin mRNA observed upon LXRβ stimulation. However SREBP-1 can activate the insulin gene expression by binding sterol regulatory elements on the insulin gene promoter as well as by serving as co-activator for BETA2/E47 [49]. Interestingly, SREBP-1 and PDX-1 may play a redundant role in controlling insulin gene expression with SREBP-1 being more efficacious under conditions of low PDX-1. In addition to these well-established LXR-target genes, expression of insulin (Ins2), glucokinase and glucose transporter 2 (GLUT2) was elevated in cells treated with T0901317. SREBP-1 is induced in β-cells by high glucose treatment and, in turn, activates expression of genes mediating cataplerosis. Mild SREBP-1 induction by hyperglycemia can be important for up-regulation of insulin secretion to adapt to the increased demand for insulin. However, long-term and strong SREBP-1 activation would eventually lead to β-cell toxicity via increased lipid accumulation [11]. The mechanisms of SREBP-1 induction under hyperglycemia in β-cells have not been studied yet. Although it is tempting that glucose itself activates LXR receptors according to Mitro *et al* [9] results.

On other hand ABC transporters may also play a pivotal role in the LXR-mediated effects on pancreas. Mice with specific inactivation of ABCA1 gene in β-cells have markedly impaired glucose tolerance and defective insulin secretion but normal insulin sensitivity [50]. Islets isolated from these mice show altered cholesterol homeostasis and impaired insulin secretion *in vitro*. The defect in insulin secretion is not due to a reduction in β-cell mass, suggesting that ABCA1 is not involved in islet development or in maintenance of β-cell mass. Rosiglitazone treatment significantly increased ABCA1 expression in the transformed rat β-cell line INS-1. The failure of rosiglitazone to improve glucose tolerance in ABCA1–Pancr/–Pancr mice suggests that specific activation of β-cell ABCA1 and subsequent reduction of islet cholesterol content is an important mechanism by which rosiglitazone improves glucose tolerance. It remains to be determined whether the effect of rosiglitazone on ABCA1 requires LXR.

LXR-agonists Increase Glucose Uptake in Adipocytes

LXR is highly expressed in adipose tissue, and its expression increases during adipogenesis and is regulated by PPARγ [37,51]. Dalen *et al* [52] have reported a strong regulation of the glucotransporter GLUT4 by LXRs. GLUT4 is expressed exclusively in tissues exhibiting insulin-stimulated glucose uptake, such as muscle, heart, and adipose tissue. The expression of GLUT4 is reduced in rodent models of insulin deficiency [53] and in adipose tissue of human obese or type-2 diabetic subjects [54], directly linking adipose expression of GLUT4 to insulin resistance. Selective ablation of GLUT4 in adipose tissue leads to decreased whole-body glucose tolerance and insulin responsiveness [55], whereas forced over-expression enhances systemic glucose clearance and insulin sensitivity [56]. Activation of LXRs in adipose tissue increases basal glucose uptake and incorporation of TGs into lipid droplets [57]. Dalen *et al* [52] have reported that the adipose tissue expression of GLUT4 is directly regulated by both LXRα and LXRβ upon ligand stimulation but that the basal expression of GLUT4 is selectively dependent on the LXRα isoform. They characterized an LXRE in the GLUT4 promoter of the human and mouse gene. They showed that GLUT4 expression is induced *in vivo* by ligand activation of LXRs after a short period of treatment. Mice treated for a short time with a PPARγ activator and/or a LXR-agonist have their expression of GLUT4 induced 3-4-fold in epididymal WAT. In muscle, a lower 1.5- and 1.6-fold induction of GLUT4 transcript was observed. In wild-type mice, the expression of GLUT4 was unchanged by insulin injection alone. In contrast, the insulin responsive transcription factor SREBP-1, was induced several-fold suggesting that GLUT4 is not normally transcriptionally regulated by insulin. Still, a synergistic induction of GLUT4 was observed with combined insulin and T0901317 treatment compared with T0901317 treatment alone. In both LXRα and LXRβ$^{-/-}$ mice, the expression of GLUT4 was induced by T0901317 treatment, with no additional effect of insulin injections. As expected, T0901317 treatment had no effect on GLUT4 expression in LXRα$^{-/-}$ β$^{-/-}$ mice, demonstrating that regulation by the LXR activator is dependent on the presence of at least one LXR isoform. The basal GLUT4 expression was slightly lower in LXRα mice compared with the other animal groups, and the slightly increased GLUT4 expression after insulin treatment was clearly absent in the LXRα mice compared with the other animal groups. This indicates that the LXRα isoform, but not the LXRβ isoform, plays a unique role for basal and insulin-regulated expression of GLUT4 in epididymal WAT.

However, the initial induction of GLUT4 expression after 24 h activation of LXRs seems to be transient and is no longer observed after prolonged treatment (one week) with a potent LXR activator. This suggests that a mechanism exists that prevents prolonged induction of GLUT4 through LXR-activation. A similar regulation has also recently been demonstrated for lipogenic genes as FAS and SREBP-1 in liver, which decline to almost normal expression levels after prolonged treatment with LXR activators (7 days). Interestingly, the expression of LXRα and SREBP-1 is similarly regulated during prolonged treatment with the LXR activator in adipose tissue, directly linking the expression level of LXRα to the induction level of GLUT4 and SREBP-1 in adipose tissue.

In adipose tissue, treatment with GW3965 [37] led to the induction of SREBP-1C and ABCA1 expression. In contrast to the effects observed in liver, expression of PGC-1 is not altered in white fat, indicating that the effects of LXR on this gene are tissue-specific. Interestingly, Laffitte *et al* [37] confirmed that LXR-agonist also stimulated expression of the insulin-sensitive glucose transporter GLUT4 in adipose tissue but had no effect on expression of GLUT1. In their study, activation of LXR led to a modest increase in expression of resistin and adiponectin but had no effect on expression of either leptin or tumor necrosis factor. The same authors measured glucose uptake in differentiated 3T3-L1 adipocytes. Treatment of the cells with the T0901317 significantly increased basal glucose uptake. Furthermore, LXR-agonist also increased insulin-stimulated glucose uptake in 3T3-L1 cells. Parallel samples processed for RNA analysis confirmed increased expression of GLUT4 mRNA in these cells under assay conditions.

LXRs seem not to play a key role in adipocyte differentiation but activation of LXRs increases TG accumulation in adipocytes [57], presumably by direct regulation of lipogenic genes as SREBP-1C and FAS. That correlates well with the finding that LXRs also regulate GLUT4, since increased glucose uptake through GLUT4 increases the substrate availability for TG synthesis.

Treatment with anti-diabetic thiazolidinediones (TZD), which are high-affinity ligands for PPARγ, normalizes the reduced adipose expression of both GLUT4 [51] and LXRα [57]. Since LXRα is a downstream target gene for PPARγ [57], the beneficial normalization of GLUT4 expression by TZD treatment might therefore actually be mediated through increased expression and activation of LXRα.

In summary LXRα expression is induced by PPARγ as a consequence of adipocyte differentiation and LXRs regulate the lipogenic transcription factor SREBP-1C, lipogenic enzymes such as FAS and stearoyl-CoA desaturase 1, the insulin-sensitive GLUT4, ApoD (a member of the lipocalin family of lipid transporters) which some polymorphisms are linked to diabetes type-2 and Spot 14 (a liver- and adipose-specific protein involved in fatty acid synthesis and lipogenesis) which has been shown to be both insulin and glucose responsive, suggesting a role for the regulation of Spot 14 in glucose metabolism [58].

LXR-agonists Affect the Glucocorticoid Pathway in Hepatocytes and Adipocytes

Increased glucocorticoid production induces obesity and type-2 diabetes via activation of intracellular GR, which mediates glucose intolerance and insulin resistance. Activation of GR itself also promotes hepatic gluconeogenesis, with an increase expression of phosphoenolpyruvate carboxykinase (PEPCK) [59]. Similarly, increased hepatic GR mRNA expression is positively correlated with the induction of insulin resistance, PEPCK mRNA expression, and hyperglycemia in diabetic db/db mice [60]. Liver specific GR knock-out mice showed reduced expression of PEPCK mRNA and are resistant to streptozotocin-induced hyperglycemia [61]. Chronic treatment of db/db mice with the LXR-agonist T0901317 reverse the induction of hepatic GR expression and attenuate the diabetic phenotype [62]. Moreover, T0901317-mediated decrease in GR gene expression is associated with the suppression of PEPCK and G6P mRNA expression thereby reducing hepatic gluconeogenesis and circulating glucose levels, all of which may contribute to preventing the development of type-2 diabetes.

11β-hydroxysteroid dehydrogenase type 1 (11β-HSD-1) converts inactive corticosteroids into biologically active corticosteroids, thereby regulating the local concentration of active glucocorticoids, such as cortisol. Mice with targeted deletion of 11β-HSD-1 are resistant to obesity- and stress-induced hyperglycemia and show attenuated hepatic up-regulation of gluconeogenic enzymes on starvation [59]. Moreover, 11β-HSD-1$^{-/-}$ mice exhibit an anti-atherogenic lipid profile with elevated levels of HDL cholesterol together with an improved glucose tolerance and lower glucose levels after refeeding, pointing to an enhanced hepatic insulin sensitivity.

11β-HSD-1 is particularly expressed in adipocytes and liver and appears to be causally linked to the development of type-2 diabetes and the metabolic syndrome. In 3T3-L1 cells and mouse embryonic fibroblasts LXR-agonists decreases mRNA expression of 11β-HSD-1 by 50%, paralleled by a significant decline in 11β-HSD-1 enzyme activity [60]. Long-term per os treatment with a synthetic LXR-agonist down-regulated 11β-HSD-1 mRNA levels by 50% in brown adipose tissue and liver of wild-type but not of LXRα/β mice and was paralleled by down-regulation of hepatic PEPCK expression [60].

Conclusion and Perpectives

Liver X Receptor (LXR) nuclear receptors modulate cholesterol and glucose metabolism in rodents and are potential drugs for the treatment of atherosclerosis and diabetes. They regulate body cholesterol transport at different levels, including absorption, excretion, catabolism, and cellular efflux. Besides these effects, they have anti-inflammatory activities which make LXR ligands attractive molecules for prevention and possibly reversion of atherosclerosis.

However these results have to be interpreted cautiously since the results here reported are in rodents and differences between species are known that may modify the pharmacological response to LXR-agonists, as for instance the absence in mice of cholesteryl ester transfer protein, a known LXR-target gene [63], and the up-regulation in mice but not humans of cholesterol 7-hydroxylase [64]. GW3965 does not increase HDL cholesterol in hamsters, and in cynomolgus monkeys but increased LDL cholesterol [65,66]. These differences underline the necessity to use human cell lines and humanized transgenic animals to select clinical candidates and to explore LXR-agonists effects in non-rodent species.

LXR-agonists have anti-diabetic effects in rodent genetic models of diabetes type-2, improving glucose tolerance and protecting pancreatic β islets. While they essentially regulate cholesterol transport via the expression of the ATP-binding cassette transporter gene family, they modulate at least in part genes of the glucose pathway via an induction of SREBP-1C which itself increases lipogenic enzymes with the risk of triglycerides deposits in the liver and other organs. It is expected than molecules which dissociate between the effect on the ABC genes as well as the NFKP pathway and the lipogenic pathway via SREBP-1C would be useful drugs for the treatment of atherosclerosis. However LXR-activation of SREBP-1 may be more problematic for their use in diabetes. LXR receptors seem to act as glucose sensor through a decrease of neoglucogenesis in the liver, an increase transport of glucose in different tissues and subsequent use in the lipogenic pathway. This appears similar to some insulin effects and many evidence indicate that insulin, glucose and LXR ligands activate common mechanisms. It will be more challenging to develop molecules in diabetes showing an acceptable balance between glucose improvement and fat deposition although capacity to activate lipogenic metabolism in the liver and other organs may differ from species to species. It should be also emphasized that the nature of the fat and reversibility of the process may have importance in the tolerance of LXR-agonists. Fat deposits are reported to decrease insulin sensitivity and be part of diabetes development, an effect not seen with LXR-agonists. It appears also that LXR-agonists have to be considered at least initially as an add-on to existing anti-diabetic drugs and more should be known of their use in combination with those drugs as well as the best treatment regimen.

Different strategies may be used to differentiate wanted and unwanted effects of LXR ligands. Targeting selective LXRβ ligand may be interesting since LXRα selective knock-out but not LXRβ knock-out mice show reduced plasma triglycerides and hepatic lipogenic gene expression [67]. However, co-crystal structures of LXR with synthetic and endogenous agonists reveal complete conservation of the ligand-binding pockets of LXRα and LXRβ [12]. Therefore, the development of LXRβ selective subtype agents may be difficult although some ligands have a preference for β subtype versus α which is not yet explained but may represent an interesting opportunity to explore. Other option would be to select compounds which are partial agonist to prevent recruitment of all pharmacological effects of full agonists or which exhibit different patterns of co-factor recruitment compared with non-selective LXR-agonists which may account for their tissue-selectivity as reported for estrogen nuclear receptor [68,69].

References

[1] P. Zimmet. Fighting the "diabesity" pandemic. *Lancet* **368** (2006) 1643.

[2] J.R. Schultz, H. Tu, A. Luk *et al.* Role of LXRs in control of lipogenesis. *Genes Dev.* **14** (2000) 2831-2838.

[3] L.J. Millatt, V. Bocher, J.C. Fruchart *et al.* Liver X receptors and the control of cholesterol homeostasis: potential therapeutic targets for the treatment of atherosclerosis. *Biochim. Biophys. Acta.* **1631** (2003) 107-118.

[4] E.G. Lund, J.G. Menke, C.P. Sparrow. Liver X receptor agonists as potential therapeutic agents for dyslipidemia and atherosclerosis. *Arterioscler. Thromb. Vasc. Biol.* **23** (2003) 1169-1177.

[5] P. Tontonoz and D.J. Mangelsdorf. Liver X receptor signaling pathways in cardiovascular disease. *Mol. Endocrinol.* **17** (2003) 985-993.

[6] S.J. Nicholls, E.M. Tuzcu, I. Sipahi *et al.* Relationship between atheroma regression and change in lumen size after infusion of apolipoprotein A-I Milano. *J. Am. Coll. Cardiol.* **47** (2006) 992-997.

[7] B.A. Janowski, P.J. Willy, T.R. Devi *et al.* An oxysterol signalling pathway mediated by the nuclear receptor LXR alpha. *Nature* **383** (1996) 728-731.

[8] A. Venkateswaran, B.A. Laffitte, S.B. Joseph *et al.* Control of cellular cholesterol efflux by the nuclear oxysterol receptor LXR alpha. *Proc. Natl. Acad. Sci. U.S.A.* **97** (2000) 12097-12102.

[9] N. Mitro, P.A. Mak, L. Vargas *et al.* The nuclear receptor LXR is a glucose sensor. *Nature* **445** (2007) 219-223.

[10] G. Cao, Y. Liang, C.L. Broderick *et al.* Antidiabetic action of a liver X receptor agonist mediated by inhibition of hepatic gluconeogenesis. *J. Biol. Chem.* **278** (2003) 1131-1136.

[11] A.M. Efanov, S. Sewing, K. Bokvist *et al.* Liver X receptor activation stimulates insulin secretion via modulation of glucose and lipid metabolism in pancreatic beta-cells. *Diabetes* **53 Suppl 3** (2004) S75-S78.

[12] J.L. Collins. Therapeutic opportunities for liver X receptor modulators. *Curr. Opin. Drug Discov. Devel.* **7** (2004) 692-702.

[13] J.J. Repa, K.E. Berge, C. Pomajzl *et al.* Regulation of ATP-binding cassette sterol transporters ABCG5 and ABCG8 by the liver X receptors alpha and beta. *J. Biol. Chem.* **277** (2002) 18793-18800.

[14] P.J. Barter. Cardioprotective effects of high-density lipoproteins: the evidence strengthens. *Arterioscler. Thromb. Vasc. Biol.* **25** (2005) 1305-1306. Comment on: *Arterioscler. Thromb. Vasc. Biol.* **25** (2005) 1325-1331; *Arterioscler. Thromb. Vasc. Biol.* **25** (2005) 1426-1432.

[15] R. Frikke-Schmidt, B.G. Nordestgaard, G.B. Jensen *et al.* Genetic variation in ABC transporter A1 contributes to HDL cholesterol in the general population. *J. Clin. Invest.* **114** (2004) 1343-1353. Comment in: *J. Clin. Invest.* **114** (2004) 1244-1247.

[16] C. Albrecht, K. Baynes, A. Sardini *et al.* Two novel missense mutations in ABCA1 result in altered trafficking and cause severe autosomal recessive HDL deficiency. *Biochim. Biophys. Acta.* **1689** (2004) 47-57.

[17] R.R. Singaraja, L.R. Brunham, H. Visscher *et al.* Efflux and atherosclerosis: the clinical and biochemical impact of variations in the ABCA1 gene. *Arterioscler. Thromb. Vasc. Biol.* **23** (2003) 1322-1332.

[18] M. Marcil, A. Brooks-Wilson, S.M. Clee *et al.* Mutations in the ABC1 gene in familial HDL deficiency with defective cholesterol efflux. *Lancet* **354** (1999) 1341-1346. Comment in: *Lancet* **354** (1999) 1402-1403.

[19] S.L. Sabol, H.B. Brewer, S. Santamarina-Fojo. The human ABCG1 gene: identification of LXR response elements that modulate expression in macrophages and liver. *J. Lipid. Res.* **46** (2005) 2151-2167.

[20] B.A. Laffitte, J.J. Repa, S.B. Joseph *et al.* LXRs control lipid-inducible expression of the apolipoprotein E gene in macrophages and adipocytes. *Proc. Natl. Acad. Sci. U.S.A.* **98** (2001) 507-512.

[21] L.K. Curtiss and W.A. Boisvert. Apolipoprotein E and atherosclerosis. *Curr. Opin. Lipidol.* **11** (2000) 243-251.

[22] P.A. Mak, B.A. Laffitte, C. Desrumaux *et al.* Regulated expression of the apolipoprotein E/C-I/C-IV/C-II gene cluster in murine and human macrophages. A critical role for nuclear liver X receptors alpha and beta. *J. Biol. Chem.* **277** (2002) 31900-31908.

[23] S.U. Naik, X. Wang, J.S. Da Silva *et al.* Pharmacological activation of liver X receptors promotes reverse cholesterol transport in vivo. *Circulation* **113** (2006) 90-97. Comment in: *Circulation* **113** (2006) 5-8.

[24] L.R. Brunham, J.K. Kruit, T.D. Pape *et al.* Tissue-specific induction of intestinal ABCA1 expression with a liver X receptor agonist raises plasma HDL cholesterol levels. *Circ. Res.* **99** (2006) 672-674.

[25] M. van Eck, I.S. Bos, W.E. Kaminski *et al.* Leukocyte ABCA1 controls susceptibility to atherosclerosis and macrophage recruitment into tissues. *Proc. Natl. Acad. Sci. U.S.A.* **99** (2002) 6298-6303.

[26] R.R. Singaraja, C. Fievet, G. Castro *et al.* Increased ABCA1 activity protects against atherosclerosis. *J. Clin. Invest.* **110** (2002) 35-42.

[27] M. Van Eck, R.R. Singaraja, D. Ye *et al.* Macrophage ATP-binding cassette transporter A1 overexpression inhibits atherosclerotic lesion progression in low-density lipoprotein receptor knockout mice. *Arterioscler. Thromb. Vasc. Biol.* **26** (2006) 929-934.

[28] N. Terasaka, A. Hiroshima, T. Koieyama *et al.* T-0901317, a synthetic liver X receptor ligand, inhibits development of atherosclerosis in LDL receptor-deficient mice. *FEBS Lett.* **536** (2003) 6-11. Comment in: *FEBS Lett.* **536** (2003) 3-5.

[29] S.B. Joseph, E. McKilligin, L. Pei *et al.* Synthetic LXR ligand inhibits the development of atherosclerosis in mice. *Proc. Natl. Acad. Sci. U.S.A.* **99** (2002) 7604-7609.

[30] N. Levin, E.D. Bischoff, C.L. Daige *et al.* Macrophage liver X receptor is required for antiatherogenic activity of LXR agonists. *Arterioscler. Thromb. Vasc. Biol.* **25** (2005) 135-142. Comment in: *Arterioscler. Thromb. Vasc. Biol.* **25** (2005) 10-11.

[31] Y. Watanabe, S. Jiang, W. Takabe *et al.* Expression of the LXRalpha protein in human atherosclerotic lesions. *Arterioscler. Thromb. Vasc. Biol.* **25** (2005) 622-627.

[32] G.K. Hansson and P. Libby. The immune response in atherosclerosis: a double-edged sword. *Nat .Rev. Immunol.* **6** (2006) 508-519.

[33] A. Castrillo, S.B. Joseph, C. Marathe *et al.* Liver X receptor-dependent repression of matrix metalloproteinase-9 expression in macrophages. *J. Biol. Chem.* **278** (2003) 10443-10449.

[34] A.J. Fowler, M.Y. Sheu, M. Schmuth *et al.* Liver X receptor activators display anti-inflammatory activity in irritant and allergic contact dermatitis models: liver-X-receptor-specific inhibition of inflammation and primary cytokine production. *J. Invest. Dermatol.* 120 (2003) 246-255. Comment in: *J. Invest. Dermatol.* **120** (2003) viii-x.

[35] D. Walcher, A. Kummel, B. Kehrle *et al.* LXR activation reduces proinflammatory cytokine expression in human CD4-positive lymphocytes. *Arterioscler. Thromb. Vasc. Biol.* **26** (2006) 1022-1028.

[36] F. Blaschke, O. Leppanen, Y. Takata *et al.* Liver X Receptor agonists suppress vascular smooth muscle cell proliferation and inhibit neointima formation in balloon-injured rat carotid arteries. *Circ. Res.* **95** (2004) 110-123.

[37] B.A. Laffitte, L.C. Chao, J. Li *et al.* Activation of liver X receptor improves glucose tolerance through coordinate regulation of glucose metabolism in liver and adipose tissue. *Proc. Natl. Acad. Sci. U.S.A.* **100** (2003) 5419-5424.

[38] I. Shimomura, Y. Bashmakov, S. Ikemoto *et al.* Insulin selectively increases SREBP-1c mRNA in the livers of rats with streptozotocin-induced diabetes. *Proc. Natl. Acad. Sci. U.S.A.* **96** (1999) 13656-13661.

[39] G. Chen, G. Liang, J. Ou *et al.* Central role for liver X receptor in insulin-mediated activation of Srebp-1c transcription and stimulation of fatty acid synthesis in liver. *Proc. Natl. Acad. Sci. U.S.A.* **101** (2004) 11245-11250.

[40] J.D. Horton, Y. Bashmakov, I. Shimomura *et al.* Regulation of sterol regulatory element binding proteins in livers of fasted and refed mice. *Proc. Natl. Acad. Sci. U.S.A.* **95** (1998) 5987-5992.

[41] D. Becard, I. Hainault, D. Azzout-Marniche *et al.* Adenovirus-mediated overexpression of sterol regulatory element binding protein-1c mimics insulin effects on hepatic gene expression and glucose homeostasis in diabetic mice. *Diabetes* **50** (2001) 2425-2430.

[42] P. Ferre, M. Foretz, D. Azzout-Marniche *et al.* Sterol-regulatory-element-binding protein 1c mediates insulin action on hepatic gene expression. *Biochem. Soc. Trans.* **29** (2001) 547-552.

[43] K. Chakravarty, P. Leahy, D. Becard *et al.* Sterol regulatory element-binding protein-1c mimics the negative effect of insulin on phosphoenolpyruvate carboxykinase (GTP) gene transcription. *J. Biol. Chem.* **276** (2001) 34816-34823.

[44] K.A. Tobin, S.M. Ulven, G.U. Schuster *et al.* Liver X receptors as insulin-mediating factors in fatty acid and cholesterol biosynthesis. *J. Biol. Chem.* **277** (2002) 10691-10697.

[45]   K.A. Tobin, H.H. Steineger, S. Alberti *et al.* Cross-talk between fatty acid and cholesterol metabolism mediated by liver X receptor-alpha. *Mol. Endocrinol.* **14** (2000) 741-752.

[46]   C.E. Juge-Aubry, E. Hammar, C. Siegrist-Kaiser *et al.* Regulation of the transcriptional activity of the peroxisome proliferator-activated receptor alpha by phosphorylation of a ligand-independent trans-activating domain. *J. Biol. Chem.* **274** (1999) 10505-10510.

[47]   H. Wang, P. Maechler, P.A. Antinozzi *et al.* The transcription factor SREBP-1c is instrumental in the development of beta-cell dysfunction. *J. Biol. Chem.* **278** (2003) 16622-16629.

[48]   H. Zitzer, W. Wente, M.B. Brenner *et al.* Sterol regulatory element-binding protein 1 mediates liver X receptor-beta-induced increases in insulin secretion and insulin messenger ribonucleic acid levels. *Endocrinology* **147** (2006) 3898-3905.

[49]   M. Amemiya-Kudo, J. Oka, T. Ide *et al.* Sterol regulatory element-binding proteins activate insulin gene promoter directly and indirectly through synergy with BETA2/E47. *J. Biol. Chem.* **280** (2005) 34577-34589.

[50]   L.R. Brunham, J.K. Kruit, T.D. Pape *et al.* Beta-cell ABCA1 influences insulin secretion, glucose homeostasis and response to thiazolidinedione treatment. *Nat. Med.* **13** (2007) 340-347.

[51]   I. Gerin, V.W. Dolinsky, J.G. Shackman *et al.* LXRbeta is required for adipocyte growth, glucose homeostasis, and beta cell function. *J. Biol. Chem.* **280** (2005) 23024-23031.

[52]   K.T. Dalen, S.M. Ulven, K. Bamberg *et al.* Expression of the insulin-responsive glucose transporter GLUT4 in adipocytes is dependent on liver X receptor alpha. *J. Biol. Chem.* **278** (2003) 48283-48291.

[53]   J. Berger, C. Biswas, P.P. Vicario *et al.* Decreased expression of the insulin-responsive glucose transporter in diabetes and fasting. *Nature* **340** (1989) 70-72.

[54]   W.T. Garvey, L. Maianu, J.A. Hancock *et al.* Gene expression of GLUT4 in skeletal muscle from insulin-resistant patients with obesity, IGT, GDM, and NIDDM. *Diabetes* **41** (1992) 465-475.

[55]   E.D. Abel, O. Peroni, J.K. Kim *et al.* Adipose-selective targeting of the GLUT4 gene impairs insulin action in muscle and liver. *Nature* **409** (2001) 729-733. Comment in: *Nature* **409** (2001) 672-673.

[56]   P.R. Shepherd, L. Gnudi, E. Tozzo *et al.* Adipose cell hyperplasia and enhanced glucose disposal in transgenic mice overexpressing GLUT4 selectively in adipose tissue. *J. Biol. Chem.* **268** (1993) 22243-22246.

[57]   L.K. Juvet, S.M. Andresen, G.U. Schuster *et al.* On the role of liver X receptors in lipid accumulation in adipocytes. *Mol. Endocrinol.* **17** (2003) 172-182.

[58]   S. Hummasti, B.A. Laffitte, M.A. Watson *et al.* Liver X receptors are regulators of adipocyte gene expression but not differentiation: identification of apoD as a direct target. *J. Lipid Res.* **45** (2004) 616-625.

[59]   J.E. Friedman, J.S. Yun, Y.M. Patel *et al.* Glucocorticoids regulate the induction phosphoenolpyruvate carboxykinase (GTP) gene transcription during diabetes. *J. Biol. Chem.* **268** (1993) 12952-12957.

[60]   Y. Liu, Y. Nakagawa, Y. Wang *et al.* Increased glucocorticoid receptor and 11{beta}-hydroxysteroid dehydrogenase type 1 expression in hepatocytes may contribute to the phenotype of type 2 diabetes in db/db mice. *Diabetes* **54** (2005) 32-40.

[61]   C. Opherk, F. Tronche, C. Kellendonk *et al.* Inactivation of the glucocorticoid receptor in hepatocytes leads to fasting hypoglycemia and ameliorates hyperglycemia in streptozotocin-induced diabetes mellitus. *Mol. Endocrinol.* **18** (2004) 1346-1353.

[62]   Y. Kotelevtsev, M.C. Holmes, A. Burchell *et al.* 11beta-hydroxysteroid dehydrogenase type 1 knockout mice show attenuated glucocorticoid-inducible responses and resist hyperglycemia on obesity or stress. *Proc. Natl. Acad. Sci. U.S.A.* **94** (1997) 14924-14929.

[63]   Y. Luo and A.R. Tall. Sterol upregulation of human CETP expression in vitro and in transgenic mice by an LXR element. *J. Clin. Invest.* **105** (2000) 513-520.

[64]   J.G. Menke, K.L. Macnaul, N.S. Hayes *et al.* A novel liver X receptor agonist establishes species differences in the regulation of cholesterol 7alpha-hydroxylase (CYP7a). *Endocrinology* **143** (2002) 2548-2558.

[65]   P.H. Groot, N.J. Pearce, J.W. Yates *et al.* Synthetic LXR agonists increase LDL in CETP species. *J. Lipid Res.* **46** (2005) 2182-2191.

[66]   B. Miao, S. Zondlo, S. Gibbs *et al.* Raising HDL cholesterol without inducing hepatic steatosis and hypertriglyceridemia by a selective LXR modulator. *J. Lipid Res.* **45** (2004) 1410-1417.

[67]   D.J. Peet, S.D. Turley, W. Ma *et al.* Cholesterol and bile acid metabolism are impaired in mice lacking the nuclear oxysterol receptor LXR alpha. *Cell* **93** (1998) 693-704.

[68]   B.S. Katzenellenbogen, I. Choi, R. Delage-Mourroux *et al.* Molecular mechanisms of estrogen action: selective ligands and receptor pharmacology. *J. Steroid Biochem. Mol. Biol.* **74** (2000) 279-285.

[69]   E.M. Quinet, D.A. Savio, A.R. Halpern *et al.* Gene-selective modulation by a synthetic oxysterol ligand of the liver X receptor. *J. Lipid Res.* **45** (2004) 1929-1942.

IOS Press, 2008

Regulation of Cardiac Energetic by the Orphan Nuclear Receptors ERRα and γ

Vincent Giguère
McGill University Health Centre, 687 Pine Avenue West, Montréal, Québec, H3A 1A1,
Canada

Abstract. Using a functional genomic approach, we have recently shown that the orphan nuclear receptors ERRα and γ coordinate a broad transcriptional program controlling energy production and utilization in the heart. In addition, both ERRs appear to be critical for normal heart function as several of their target genes are known to be associated with human cardiomyopathies. The ability to regulate the activity of ERRα and/or ERRγ using synthetic ligands suggests the potential for new therapeutic approaches to prevent and manage cardiovascular diseases.

Keywords. Chromatin immunoprecipitation, estrogen-related receptors, mitochondria, PGC-1

Introduction

Nuclear receptors are transcription factors that play critical roles in development, reproduction and homeostasis through the control of specific gene networks. The superfamily of nuclear receptors is comprised of both classic and orphan receptors. Classic receptors bind to and are activated by high-affinity lipophilic ligands whose discoveries preceded that of the receptors (e.g. estradiol, testosterone, cortisol). On the other hand, orphan nuclear receptors are receptor-like proteins with no associated ligands at the time of their discovery [1]. The unexpected identification of these putative receptors suggested that ligand-based response systems controlling diverse biological functions remained to be found [2]. This hypothesis was validated by the subsequent identification of retinoic acids, prostaglandins, bile acids, hydroxycholesterols, fatty acids, phospholipids as well as various drugs and other xenobiotic agents as orphan nuclear receptor ligands. In addition, genetic studies in animal models and in human showed that orphan nuclear receptors influence reproduction, nutrition, carbohydrate and lipid metabolism, energy balance, inflammation and innate host defense, and have been associated with common diseases such as diabetes, obesity, atherosclerosis, osteoporosis, Parkinson's and cancer. Notably, structural and functional studies showed most orphan receptors to be attractive, "druggable" targets [reviewed in 3]. The research interest of our laboratory has been centered on the investigation of the biological roles of a subfamily of orphan nuclear receptors, referred to as the estrogen-related receptor (ERR). Recent work by us and other groups indicates that the ERRs may play important roles in metabolic control, fat absorption, mitochondrial biogenesis, adaptive thermogenesis, cardiovascular disease, osteoporosis and macrophage function in host resistance. The review will focus on our recent discovery that the ERRs act as master regulators of cardiac energy production and utilization.

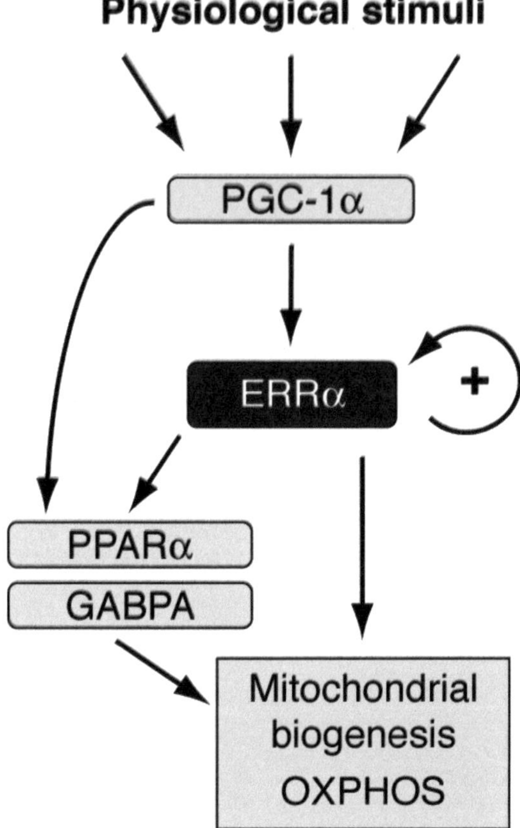

Figure 1. ERRα acts a conduit for PGC-1α in the control of energy metabolism.
PGC-1α expression is up-regulated in response to physiological stimuli such as exposure to cold, fasting or exercise. PGC-1α then binds to and increases the transcriptional activity of ERRα. In a feed forward loop, ERRα increases it own expression and that of other transcription factors such as PPARα and GABPA (NRF-2). Together, these factors regulate genes involved in mitochondrial biogenesis and oxidative phosphorylation (OXPHOS).

1. Cardiac Energetics

In order to stay healthy and function as a dependable pump, the heart must produce enough ATP to maintain intracellular Ca^{2+} homeostasis for contraction. Indeed, the progression to heart failure is always accompanied by a gradual reduction in the capacity for ATP-generation [reviewed in 4,5]. The adult heart utilizes oxidation of both fatty acids (FAs) and glucose in mitochondria to generate the ATP required for its specialized functions. Because energy demand and energy substrate availability are constantly changing in response to environmental cues, the ATP-generating machinery must be able to adapt rapidly and efficiently to these changes. In particular, the heart must be able to switch between sources of energy in response to the physiological needs of the individual, and to estimate the cellular energy status of cardiac cells [6,7]. This metabolic flexibility is mediated by allosteric controls and post-translation modifications for short-term alterations as well as changes in the expression of metabolic genes for long-term regulation. Furthermore, because ATP-synthesis is tightly matched with demand, coordinated regulation of ATP-generating and utilization pathways is often observed during development and in response to physiologic and pathophysiologic changes. Thus, this complex regulatory network requires the coordinated transcriptional regulation of genes encoding proteins implicated in FA and glucose uptake, handling of the metabolic intermediates, FA β-oxidation (FAO) and pyruvate oxidation complexes, as well as the common oxidative pathways of tricarboxylic acid cycle (TCA), electron transport complex (ETC) and oxidative phosphorylation (OXPHOS). In addition, the expression of proteins involved in energy utilization (mitochondrial/cytoplasmic ADP-ATP exchange, phosphate transfer, fuel-sensing, and ATPases involved in calcium uptake and actomyosin crossbridging) have also to be regulated in unison. Although several transcription factors have been shown to play essential roles in heart development and the control of energy metabolism [8-10], none of these factors have been shown to assimilate the control of energy generation and utilization in a comprehensive manner.

2. The ERRs and PGC-1 Co-activators: An "Energetic" Relationship

ERRα and β were the first orphan nuclear receptors identified through a search for genes encoding proteins related to the estrogen receptor (ER) [2]. A third member of the family, ERRγ, was identified a decade later [11-14]. Consequently, initial studies on ERRs focused on their potential involvement in estrogen signaling [reviewed in 15]. While the ERRs can indeed function in classic estrogen-responsive systems such as bones and breast cancer cells [16,17], it now appears that their primary and most essential task is to act as regulators of energy metabolism. The first evidence that the ERRs could be involved in the control of energy metabolism consisted in the finding that a consensus binding site for ERRα was embedded within an essential regulatory element located in the promoter of the medium-chain acyl-coenzyme A dehydrogenase gene (MCAD, *Acadm*) [18,19]. This enzyme catalyzes the initial step of the mitochondrial fatty acid β-oxidation pathway, and its level of expression helps to determine the metabolic potential of a tissue. The second relevant observation was the finding that despite their structural homology with the ER, the ERRs are not activated by estrogens or any other natural compounds. Instead, the transcriptional activity of the ERRs is dependent on interactions with co-activators, in particular PGC-1α and PGC-1β [20-24]. The functional relationship between the ERRs and PGC-1 co-activators was of significant interest as these co-activators were known to play essential roles in mitochondrial biogenesis and gluconeogenesis in the liver [reviewed in 25]. Subsequent studies showed that PGC-1α can induce the expression of ERRα when introduced into cells in culture [23], and we showed that a polymorphic autoregulatory hormone response element present in the promoter of the gene encoding human ERRα was responsible for this induction [22,26]. The two genes are indeed co-expressed in tissues with high energy demands, and are co-induced in a tissue-specific fashion in response to physiological stresses such as fasting, exposure to cold and exercise [18,23,27-29]. ERRγ and PGC-1β are also highly expressed in mitochondria-rich tissues with high energy needs such as the heart and brown adipose tissue, and to a lesser extent in skeletal muscle, liver and white adipose tissue [11,30]. PGC-1β expression is elevated in the liver during fasting and in response to short-term high-fat feeding of mice [31]. It was also observed that over-expression of PGC-1α leads to the expression of several genes involved in OXPHOS, and that the promoters of these genes often contain putative binding sites for ERRα [32,33]. These studies also showed that inhibiting ERRα activity by using an siRNA or the small inverse agonist XCT790 in cultured cells reduced the ability of PGC-1α to induce respiration and mitochondrial biogenesis. Similarly, it was shown that expression in HepG2 cells of a modified PGC-1α protein able only to recognize the three ERRs led to an increase in the expression of OXPHOS genes [34]. These results suggested that the ERRs may indeed act as the major conduits for PGC-1α and β action in the control of mitochondrial biogenesis and energy metabolism (Figure 1).

3. Exploring the Role of ERRα and γ Using Mouse Genetics

3.1. ERRα, β and γ Null Mice

To understand the *in vivo* function of the ERRs, we and our collaborators generated and analyzed ERRα (*Esrra^{-/-}*), ERRβ (*Esrrb^{-/-}*) and ERRγ (*Esrrg^{-/-}*) null mice. The *Esrrb^{-/-}* mice were studied first, and our phenotypic analysis showed ERRβ to be essential for early placentation and thus are embryonic lethal [35]. Although tetraploid rescue experiments showed that the *Esrrb^{-/-}* embryos develop normally and can produce adult animals [35,36], studies in adult mice have yet to be performed on a large scale for practical reasons. In contrast, phenotypic analysis of the *Esrra^{-/-}* mice showed them to be viable and fertile with no gross anatomical alterations, with the exception of reduced body weight and peripheral fat deposits [37]. The *Esrra^{-/-}* mice also showed altered expression of genes involved in lipid metabolism and OXPHOS in several tissues, including white adipose tissue, muscle and small intestine [37-39]. Although the changes observed in the expression of metabolic genes in these tissues should, in theory, lead the mice to burn less fat and spend less energy, the mice are paradoxically lean and resistant to diet-induced obesity [37]. These observations suggest a more complex and tissue-specific role for ERRα in the control of energy metabolism in the whole animal, thus requiring more subtle genetic models and phenotypic analyses. The *Esrrg^{-/-}* mice have been recently produced in the laboratory of Ron Evans in La Jolla [W. Alaynick, personal communication]. The hearts of ERRγ null mice fail at birth, an event that is coincident with the required increase in cardiac oxidative capacity and shift from reliance on glucose metabolism to oxidation of fats for energy.

3.2. ERRα Regulates Mitochondrial Biogenesis and Adaptive Thermogenesis

Brown adipose tissue has a very high mitochondrial content and expresses high levels of ERRα, PGC-1α and PGC-1β [18,19,29,30]. Brown adipose tissue produces heat and promotes energy expenditure in response to cold temperatures and subsequent activation of the sympathetic nervous system. Failure to induce the expression of PGC-1α or uncoupling protein-1 and/or deficiency in mitochondrial oxidative capacity lead to defective thermogenesis [40,41]. The role of ERRα in brown adipose tissue mitochondrial biogenesis and adaptive thermogenesis *in vivo* was recently investigated [42]. This work showed that in the absence of ERRα, mice display a reduced mitochondrial mass in brown adipose tissue and impaired thermogenic capacity in response to cold temperatures, leading to hypothermia and slower recovery to a normal body temperature. These findings showed that ERRα is indeed essential for the organism in situations of high energy demand and suggest that defects in ERRα function could contribute to pathological states caused by mitochondrial dysfunction.

4. ERRα and γ Control Cardiac Energetic and Contractile Functions

4.1. ERRα Is Required for Cardiac Adaptation to Pressure Overlaod

As introduced above, the heart is a specialized tissue with constant high energy demands, and progressive decline in the activity of mitochondrial respiratory pathways leading to reduced capacity for ATP-production is a feature of cardiac hypertrophy and heart failure [4]. The vast majority of ATP-generation in the heart is performed in mitochondria via oxidation of fatty acids and glucose. Also noted above, ERRα expression corresponds to that of PGC-1α in the heart, and its levels are increased via introduction of PGC-1α in cardiac myocytes [39]. Mainly through classic investigation of candidate genes, the ERRα/PGC-1α complex was shown to directly regulate genes that encode mitochondrial enzymes such as MCAD (*Acadm*), cytochrome c (*Cycs*), ATP-synthase (*Atp5b*) and monoamine oxidase (*Maoa*) as well as factors controlling mitochondrial biogenesis such as PPARα (*Ppara*) and NRF-2 (Gapba), and PDK4 (*Pdk4*), a kinase directing substrate utilization [18,19,32,33,39,43,44]. To learn more about the role of ERRα in the heart, alterations in cardiac energy metabolism in ERRα null mice during pathologic cardiac remodeling were monitored. In collaboration with Dan Kelly's group in St-Louis and Janice Huss at City of Hope, our groups found that the hearts of ERRα null mice subjected to transverse aortic constriction to induce pressure overload were hypertrophied to a greater extant than that of wild-type mice, and that phosphocreatine and ATP-levels were significantly depleted in ERRα null hearts after β-adrenergic stimulation. It is interesting to note that a similar phenotype was observed in PGC-1α null mice [45]. Thus, given the fact that the ERRα null hearts have reduced energetic levels, these results suggest once again that the ERRα/PGC-1α complex regulates genes involved in energy metabolism.

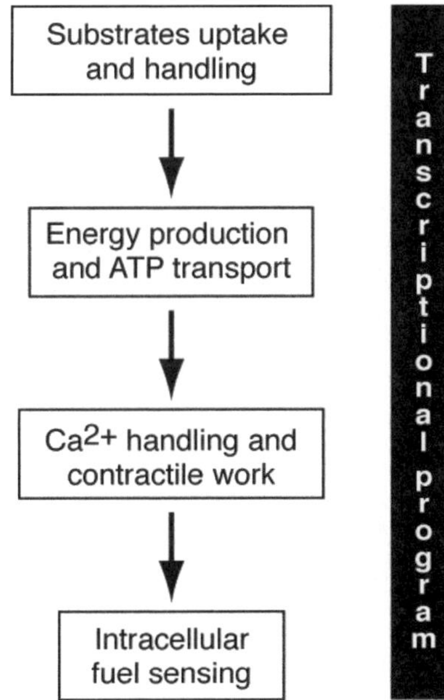

Figure 2. Global regulation of cardiac functions by orphan nuclear receptors ERRα and γ.
Genome-wide location analysis indicates that ERRα and γ regulate a broad genetic program involved in every aspect of heart function.

4.2. Location Analysis of ERRα and ERRγ Binding in the Mouse Heart

In order to obtain a more accurate and global view of the role of ERRα as a transcription factor in the heart, as well as to begin an investigation of the role of ERRγ in this tissue where it is also expressed at high levels, we recently used a combination of genome-wide location analysis (ChIP-on-chip) and expression profiling in normal and ERRα null mouse heart to identify a network of overlapping targets of both ERRα and γ [46]. We found that ERRα and γ, working as non-obligatory heterodimers, bind to a common set of promoters involved in all aspect of cardiac functions, including uptake of energy substrates, production and transport of ATP across the mitochondrial membranes, cytosolic fuel-sensing as well as calcium handling and contractile work. In agreement with the recognized role of the ERRs in the regulation of mitochondrial functions, a large number of target genes encode proteins involved in OXPHOS and the tricarboxylic acid cycle. Other ERR target genes identified proteins playing a role in glucose and fatty acid metabolism such as PDK4, GLUT12, HK2, H-FABP and LDHB. Other target genes encode proteins involved in specific muscle function such as calsequestrin, cypher and telethonin, or transcriptional gene regulation such as p53, retinoic acid receptor α and the co-activators AMY-1 and SKIIP. Finally, computational prediction made with more than 300 ERR target promoters supported by functional analyses identified STAT-3 as a transcription factor that collaborates with the ERRs in the regulation of a subset of genes devoid of recognizable consensus ERR response elements. Interestingly, *Pias3*, the gene encoding protein inhibitor of activated STAT 3 (PIAS3), is also a direct target of ERRα in this tissue, suggesting the existence of a tightly controlled transcriptional regulatory network [46]. The role of ERRγ in controlling OXPHOS as well as structural genes important for normal newborn heart function was validated by ChIP-on-chip and standard ChIP experiments performed in our laboratory.

5. ERR Target Genes Are Linked to Cardiomyopathies

The biological significance of the ERR target genes in the mouse heart is further exemplified by the knowledge that a large number of these genes have been linked to specific cardiac phenotypes in various mouse models and/or cardiomyopathies in humans. *Ldbh*, *Phc1*, *Rara*, *Slc25a4*, *Tcap* and *Trp53* have all been associated with dilated cardiomyopathies and other cardiac dysfunctions [47-54] while mutations in *Ckm* and *Ckmt2* have been linked with left ventricular hypertrophy [55,56].

6. Conclusion

The work described here, using functional genomics and genetically altered mouse models, highlighted unanticipated biological roles and mechanisms of action for the ERRs in the heart. More importantly, these results suggest that potential synthetic ERR ligands [57-62], especially those targeting ERRγ, could be used to control myocardial energy levels and manage associated cardiomyopathies.

References

[1]   V. Giguère. Orphan nuclear receptors: from gene to function. *Endocr. Rev.* **20** (1999) 689-725.

[2]   V. Giguère, N. Yang, P. Segui *et al.* Identification of a new class of steroid hormone receptors. *Nature* **331** (1988) 91-94.

[3]   R. Mohan and R.A. Heyman. Orphan nuclear receptor modulators. *Curr. Top Med. Chem.* **3** (2003) 1637-1647.

[4]   J.M. Huss and D.P. Kelly. Mitochondrial energy metabolism in heart failure: a question of balance. *J. Clin. Invest.* **115** (2005) 547-555.

[5]   J.S. Ingwall and R.G. Weiss. Is the failing heart energy starved? On using chemical energy to support cardiac function. *Circ. Res.* **95** (2004) 135-145.

[6]   H. Taegtmeyer, L. Golfman, S. Sharma *et al.* Linking gene expression to function: metabolic flexibility in the normal and diseased heart. *Ann. N.Y. Acad. Sci.* **1015** (2004) 202-213.

[7]   H. Taegtmeyer, C.R. Wilson, P. Razeghi *et al.* Metabolic energetics and genetics in the heart. *Ann. N.Y. Acad. Sci.* **1047** (2005) 208-218.

[8]   E.N. Olson. Gene regulatory networks in the evolution and development of the heart. *Science* **313** (2006) 1922-1927.

[9]   J.M. Huss and D.P. Kelly. Nuclear receptor signaling and cardiac energetics. *Circ. Res.* **95** (2004) 568-578.

[10]   R.C. Scarpulla. Nuclear control of respiratory gene expression in mammalian cells. *J. Cell Biochem.* **97** (2006) 673-683.

[11]   H. Hong, L. Yang, M.R. Stallcup. Hormone-independent transcriptional activation and coactivator binding by novel orphan nuclear receptor ERR3. *J. Biol. Chem.* **274** (1999) 22618-22626.

[12]   J.D. Eudy, S. Yao, M.D. Weston *et al.* Isolation of a gene encoding a novel member of the nuclear receptor superfamily from the critical region of Usher syndrome type IIa at 1q41. *Genomics* **50** (1998) 382-384.

[13]   D.J. Heard, P.L. Norby, J. Holloway *et al.* Human ERRgamma, a third member of the estrogen receptor-related receptor (ERR) subfamily of orphan nuclear receptors: tissue-specific isoforms are expressed during development and in the adult. *Mol. Endocrinol.* **14** (2000) 382-392.

[14]   F. Chen, Q. Zhang, T. McDonald *et al.* Identification of two hERR2-related novel nuclear receptors utilizing bioinformatics and inverse PCR. *Gene* **228** (1999) 101-109.

[15]   V. Giguère. To ERR in the estrogen pathway. *Trends Endocrinol. Metab.* **13** (2002) 220-225.

[16]   J.B. Barry and V. Giguère. Epidermal growth factor-induced signaling in breast cancer cells results in selective target gene activation by orphan nuclear receptor estrogen-related receptor alpha. *Cancer Res.* **65** (2005) 6120-6129.

[17]   E. Bonnelye and J.E. Aubin. Estrogen receptor-related receptor alpha: a mediator of estrogen response in bone. *J. Clin. Endocrinol. Metab.* **90** (2005) 3115-3121.

[18]   R. Sladek, J.A. Bader, V. Giguère. The orphan nuclear receptor estrogen-related receptor alpha is a transcriptional regulator of the human medium-chain acyl coenzyme A dehydrogenase gene. *Mol. Cell. Biol.* **17** (1997) 5400-5409.

[19]   R.B. Vega and D.P. Kelly. A role for estrogen-related receptor alpha in the control of mitochondrial fatty acid beta-oxidation during brown adipocyte differentiation. *J. Biol. Chem.* **272** (1997) 31693-31699.

[20]   J.M. Huss, R.P. Kopp, D.P. Kelly. Peroxisome proliferator-activated receptor coactivator-1alpha (PGC-1alpha) coactivates the cardiac-enriched nuclear receptors estrogen-related receptor-alpha and -gamma. Identification of novel leucine-rich interaction motif within PGC-1alpha. *J. Biol. Chem.* **277** (2002) 40265-40274.

[21]   Y. Kamei, H. Ohizumi, Y. Fujitani *et al.* PPARgamma coactivator 1beta/ERR ligand 1 is an ERR protein ligand, whose expression induces a high-energy expenditure and antagonizes obesity. *Proc. Natl. Acad. Sci. U.S.A.* **100** (2003) 12378-12383.

[22]   J. Laganière, G.B. Tremblay, C.R. Dufour *et al.* A polymorphic autoregulatory hormone response element in the human estrogen-related receptor alpha (ERRalpha) promoter dictates peroxisome proliferator-activated receptor gamma coactivator-1alpha control of ERRalpha expression. *J. Biol. Chem.* **279** (2004) 18504-18510.

[23]   S.N. Schreiber, D. Knutti, K. Brogli *et al.* The transcriptional coactivator PGC-1 regulates the expression and activity of the orphan nuclear receptor estrogen-related receptor alpha (ERRalpha). *J. Biol. Chem.* **278** (2003) 9013-9018.

[24]   J.B. Barry, J. Laganière, V. Giguère. A single nucleotide in an estrogen-related receptor alpha site can dictate mode of binding and peroxisome proliferator-activated receptor gamma coactivator 1alpha activation of target promoters. *Mol. Endocrinol.* **20** (2006) 302-310.

[25]   J. Lin, C. Handschin, B.M. Spiegelman. Metabolic control through the PGC-1 family of transcription coactivators. *Cell Metab.* **1** (2005) 361-370.

[26]   N. Laflamme, S. Giroux, J.C. Loredo-Osti *et al.* A frequent regulatory variant of the estrogen-related receptor alpha gene associated with BMD in French-Canadian premenopausal women. *J. Bone Miner. Res.* **20** (2005) 938-944.

[27]   R. Cartoni, B. Léger, M.B. Hock *et al.* Mitofusins 1/2 and ERRalpha expression are increased in human skeletal muscle after physical exercise. *J. Physiol.* **567** (2005) 349-358.

[28]   M. Ichida, S. Nemoto, T. Finkel. Identification of a specific molecular repressor of the peroxisome proliferator-activated receptor gamma Coactivator-1alpha (PGC-alpha). *J. Biol. Chem.* **277** (2002) 50991-50995.

[29]   P. Puigserver, Z. Wu, C.W. Park *et al.* A cold-inducible coactivator of nuclear receptors linked to adaptive thermogenesis. *Cell* **92** (1998) 829-839.

[30]   J. Lin, P. Puigserver, J. Donovan *et al.* 2002 Peroxisome proliferator-activated receptor gamma coactivator 1beta (PGC-1beta), a novel PGC-1-related transcription coactivator associated with host cell factor. *J. Biol. Chem.* **277** (2002) 1645-1648.

[31]   J. Lin, R. Yang, P.T. Tarr *et al.* Hyperlipidemic effects of dietary saturated fats mediated through PGC-1beta coactivation of SREBP. *Cell* **120** (2005) 261-273.

[32]   V.K. Mootha, C. Handschin, D. Arlow *et al.* ERRalpha and GABPAa/b specify PGC-1alpha-dependent oxidative phosphorylation gene expression that is altered in diabetic muscle. *Proc. Natl. Acad. Sci. U.S.A.* **101** (2004) 6570-6575. Erratum in: *Proc. Natl. Acad. Sci. U.S.A.* **102** (2005) 10405.

[33]   S.N. Schreiber, R. Emter, M.B. Hock *et al.* The estrogen-related receptor alpha (ERRalpha) functions in PPARgamma coactivator 1alpha (PGC-1alpha)-induced mitochondrial biogenesis. *Proc. Natl. Acad. Sci. U.S.A.* **101** (2004) 6472-6477.

[34]   S. Gaillard, L.L. Grasfeder, C.L. Haeffele *et al.* Receptor-selective coactivators as tools to define the biology of specific receptor-coactivator pairs. *Mol. Cell* **24** (2006) 797-803.

[35]   J. Luo, R. Sladek, J.A. Bader *et al.* Placental abnormalities in mouse embryos lacking orphan nuclear receptor ERR-beta. *Nature* **388** (1997) 778-782.

[36]   K. Mitsunaga, K. Araki, H. Mizusaki *et al.* Loss of PGC-specific expression of the orphan nuclear receptor ERR-beta results in reduction of germ cell number in mouse embryos. *Mech. Dev.* **121** (2004) 237-246.

[37]   J. Luo, R. Sladek, J. Carrier *et al.* Reduced fat mass in mice lacking orphan nuclear receptor estrogen-related receptor alpha. *Mol. Cell. Biol.* **23** (2003) 7947-7956.

[38]   J.C. Carrier, G. Deblois, C. Champigny *et al.* Estrogen related-receptor alpha (ERRalpha) is a transcriptional regulator of apolipoprotein A-IV and controls lipid handling in the intestine. *J. Biol. Chem.* **279** (2004) 52052-52058.

[39]   J.M. Huss, I.P. Torra, B. Staels *et al.* Estrogen-related receptor alpha directs peroxisome proliferator-activated receptor alpha signaling in the transcriptional control of energy metabolism in cardiac and skeletal muscle. *Mol. Cell. Biol.* **24** (2004) 9079-9091.

[40]   T.C. Leone, J.J. Lehman, B.N. Finck *et al.* PGC-1alpha deficiency causes multi-system energy metabolic derangements: muscle dysfunction, abnormal weight control and hepatic steatosis. *PLoS Biol.* **3** (2005) e101.

[41]   J. Lin, P.H. Wu, P.T. Tarr *et al.* Defects in adaptive energy metabolism with CNS-linked hyperactivity in PGC-1alpha null mice. *Cell* **119** (2004) 121-135. Comment in: *Cell* **119** (2004) 5-7.

[42]   J.A. Villena, M.B. Hock, W.Y. Chang *et al.* Orphan nuclear receptor estrogen-related receptor alpha is essential for adaptive thermogenesis. *Proc. Natl. Acad. Sci. U.S.A.* **104** (2007) 1418-1423.

[43]   A.R. Wende, J.M. Huss, P.J. Schaeffer *et al.* PGC-1alpha coactivates PDK4 gene expression via the orphan nuclear receptor ERRalpha: a mechanism for transcriptional control of muscle glucose metabolism. *Mol. Cell. Biol.* **25** (2005) 10684-10694.

[44]   M. Araki and K. Motojima. Identification of ERRalpha as a specific partner of PGC-1alpha for the activation of PDK4 gene expression in muscle. *FEBS J.* **273** (2006) 1669-1680.

[45]   Z. Arany, M. Novikov, S. Chin *et al.* Transverse aortic constriction leads to accelerated heart failure in mice lacking PPAR-gamma coactivator 1alpha. *Proc. Natl. Acad. Sci. U.S.A.* **103** (2006) 10086-10091.

[46]   C.R. Dufour, B.J. Wilson, J.M. Huss *et al.* Gemone-wide orchestration of cardiac functions by the orphan nuclear receptors ERRalpha and gamma. *Cell Metab.* **5** (2007) 345-356.

[47]   D. Cesselli, I. Jakoniuk, L. Barlucchi *et al.* Oxidative stress-mediated cardiac cell death is a major determinant of ventricular dysfunction and failure in dog dilated cardiomyopathy. *Circ. Res.* **89** (2001) 279-286. Comment in: *Circ. Res.* **89** (2001) 198-200.

[48]   H. Morita, J. Seidman, C.E. Seidman. Genetic causes of human heart failure. *J. Clin. Invest.* **115** (2005) 518-526.

[49]   B.H. Graham, K.G. Waymire, B. Cottrell *et al.* A mouse model for mitochondrial myopathy and cardiomyopathy resulting from a deficiency in the heart/muscle isoform of the adenine nucleotide translocator. *Nat. Genet.* **16** (1997) 226-234.

[50]   P. Kastner, N. Messaddeq, M. Mark *et al.* Vitamin A deficiency and mutations of RXRalpha, RXRbeta and RARalpha lead to early differentiation of embryonic ventricular cardiomyocytes. *Development* **124** (1997) 4749-4758.

[51]   H. Koga, Y. Kaji, K. Nishii *et al.* Overexpression of Polycomb-group gene rae28 in cardiomyocytes does not complement abnormal cardiac morphogenesis in mice lacking rae28 but causes dilated cardiomyopathy. *Lab. Invest.* **82** (2002) 375-385.

[52]   M. Vatta, B. Mohapatra, S. Jimenez *et al.* Mutations in Cypher/ZASP in patients with dilated cardiomyopathy and left ventricular non-compaction. *J. Am. Coll. Cardiol.* **42** (2003) 2014-2027. Comment in: *J. Am. Coll. Cardiol.* **44** (2004) 1139: author reply 1139-1140.

[53]   T. Arimura, T. Hayashi, H. Terada *et al.* A Cypher/ZASP mutation associated with dilated cardiomyopathy alters the binding affinity to protein kinase C. *J. Biol. Chem.* **279** (2004) 6746-6752.

[54]   M. Sano, T. Minamino, H. Toko *et al.* p53-induced inhibition of Hif-1 causes cardiac dysfunction during pressure overload. *Nature* **446** (2007) 444-448.

[55]   M. Fountoulakis, E. Soumaka, K. Rapti *et al.* Alterations in the heart mitochondrial proteome in a desmin null heart failure model. *J. Mol. Cell. Cardiol.* **38** (2005) 461-474.

[56]   M. Nahrendorf, M. Spindler, K. Hu *et al.* Creatine kinase knockout mice show left ventricular hypertrophy and dilatation, but unaltered remodeling post-myocardial infarction. *Cardiovasc. Res.* **65** (2005) 419-427.

[57]   G.B. Tremblay, D. Bergeron, V. Giguère. 4-Hydroxytamoxifen is an isoform-specific inhibitor of orphan estrogen-receptor-related (ERR) nuclear receptors beta and gamma. *Endocrinology* **142** (2001) 4572-4575.

[58]   G.B. Tremblay, T. Kunath, D. Bergeron *et al.* Diethylstilbestrol regulates trophoblast stem cell differentiation as a ligand of orphan nuclear receptor ERR beta. *Genes Dev.* **15** (2001) 833-838.

[59]   E.Y. Chao, J.L. Collins, S. Gaillard *e al.* Structure-guided synthesis of tamoxifen analogs with improved selectivity for the orphan ERRgamma. *Bioorg. Med. Chem. Lett.* **16** (2006) 821-824.

[60]   D.D. Yu and B.M. Forman. 2005 Identification of an agonist ligand for estrogen-related receptors ERRbeta/gamma. *Bioorg. Med. Chem. Lett.* **15** (2005) 1311-1313.

[61]   P. Coward, D. Lee, M.V. Hull *et al.* 4-Hydroxytamoxifen binds to and deactivates the estrogen-related receptor gamma. *Proc. Natl. Acad. Sci. U.S.A.* **98** (2001) 8880-8884.

[62]   P.J. Willy, I.R. Murray, J. Qian *et al.* Regulation of PPARgamma coactivator 1alpha (PGC-1alpha) signaling by an estrogen-related receptor alpha (ERRalpha) ligand. *Proc. Natl. Acad. Sci. U.S.A.* **101** (2004) 8912-8917.

Nuclear Receptors as Molecular Targets for Cardiometabolic and Central Nervous System Diseases   43
J.L. Junien and B. Staels (Eds.)
IOS Press, 2008

FXR and Bile Acids: Critical Modulators of Metabolism

Peter A. Edwards[a,b,c] and Yanqiao Zhang[a,b]
[a]*Department of Biological Chemistry, University of California at Los Angeles, 33-257 CHS, 10833 Le Conte Ave., Los Angeles, CA 90095, USA*
[b]*Department of Medicine, University of California at Los Angeles, 33-257 CHS, 10833 Le Conte Ave., Los Angeles, CA 90095, USA*
[c]*The Molecular Biology Institute, University of California at Los Angeles, CA 90095, USA*

Abstract. Bile acids are the natural agonists for the nuclear receptor Farnesoid X Receptor (FXR). Studies utilizing natural and synthetic FXR-agonists and FXR null mice indicate that FXR controls numerous metabolic pathways, including those involved in bile acid, lipid and glucose homeostasis. In addition, FXR functions to control bacterial growth in the intestine, gallstone formation, hepatic regeneration and tumorogenesis. Thus, FXR may represent a novel target for pharmaceutical intervention that may influence various metabolic disorders or diseases.

Keywords. Bile acids, enterohepatic circulation, glucose, lipoproteins

1. Introduction

The mammalian Farnesoid X Receptor (FXRα, NR1H4) was first cloned in 1995 [1,2]. The finding that the amino-acid sequence is conserved from teleost fish to humans suggests a common function across many species. FXR is a member of the nuclear receptor (NR) superfamily that contains 48 human and 49 rodent members. Most NRs are ligand-activated transcriptional factors that bind to specific DNA sequences (response elements) and activate transcription of target genes. Some NRs are considered orphans because a ligand that binds to the ligand-binding domain has yet to be identified, or they may be constitutively active in the absence of any ligand. A few NRs, for example small heterodimer partner (SHP; NR0B2), do not bind directly to DNA but instead bind to and alter the activity of other DNA-binding transcription factors [3]. Natural agonists identified to date tend to be small lipophylic compounds; they include steroid hormones, thyroid hormone, 1,25-dihydroxyvitamin D3, fatty acids, oxysterols, retinoic acids, phospholipids and bile acids.

FXRα is expressed at high levels in the liver, intestine, kidney and adrenal gland [1,2,4,5]. Low levels of FXR are reported in white adipose tissue and heart. However, the functional significance of the low levels of FXR in these latter two issues is unknown [4,6,7]. FXR binds to FXR response elements (FXREs) as a heterodimer with Retinoid X Receptor (RXR, NR2B1). The DNA sequence corresponding to an FXRE usually contains two copies of a consensus sequence (AGGTCA) arranged as an <u>i</u>nverted <u>r</u>epeat separated by one nucleotide (IR1), an <u>e</u>verted <u>r</u>epeat separated by 8 nucleotides (ER8) or a <u>d</u>irect <u>r</u>epeat separated by four nucleotides (DR4) [8,9]. FXREs have been identified in the proximal promoters of target genes, many kilo-base pairs from the transcriptional start site and in intronic regions. In rare cases FXR has been shown to bind to DNA as a monomer [10].

The readers are referred to the many excellent recent reviews on FXR and/or bile acid metabolism [8-13].

2. FXR-agonists

The original natural agonist for FXR was thought to be the 15 carbon isoprenoid alcohol, farnesol (hence the name FXR) [1]. However farnesol is a very weak agonist for FXR. A key breakthrough came in 1999 when bile acids were shown to bind to FXR and to be far more potent agonists at physiological concentrations [14-16]. Active bile acids include chenodeoxycholic acid (CDCA), lithocholic acid (LCA), deoxycholic acid (DCA) and cholic acid (CA) (Figure 1). Although androsterone, an intermediate in steroid biosynthesis, has been shown to function as a weak FXR-agonist, it is unclear whether such activation is of physiological importance [17].

Studies over the last few years have shown that bile acids not only activate FXR, but also activate the pregnane X receptor (PXR), vitamin D receptor (VDR) and the constitutive androstane receptor (CAR) [12] (Figure 1). In addition, bile acids regulate c-Jun N-terminal kinase (JNK) cascade and the mitogen-activated protein kinase pathway, independent of nuclear receptor activation. More recent studies have shown that bile acids also activate a G-protein coupled receptor Gpbar (G-protein bile acid activated receptor)/TGR5 that is expressed on the cell surface of many tissues including brown adipose tissue and the gall bladder (Figure 1) [18]. Thus, bile acids are capable of activating numerous signaling pathways (reviewed in [12]).

Because bile acids activate so many NRs it was important to identify FXR-specific agonists to allow facile separation of FXR-dependent and FXR-independent pathways; such agonists include GW4064 [19], fexaramine [20], AGN34 [21] and 6α-ethyl-chenodeoxycholic acid (6-ECDCA) [22] (Figure 1). In addition, the generation of FXR-deficient mice [23] has allowed investigators to distinguish between FXR-dependent and -independent pathways.

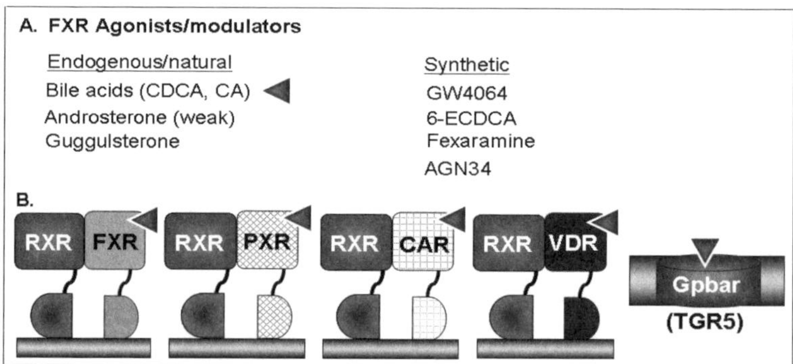

Figure 1. FXR-agonists and modulators. A) Endogenous/natural and synthetic FXR-agonists are shown. B) Bile acids can activate both nuclear receptors (FXR, PXR, CAR and VDR) and a G-protein coupled receptor (Gpbar, TGR5).

3. FXR and the Regulation of Bile Acid Metabolism

The liver is the sole site of catabolism of cholesterol to bile acids (Figure 2). For decades the sole function of bile acids was thought to be the dispersion of lipids in the intestinal lumen in order to facilitate enzymatic digestion of dietary lipids, a process that precedes lipid absorption. It has also been known for decades that approximately 95% of the bile acids secreted into the intestine are actively reabsorbed in the distal ileum and returned to the liver in a process termed the enterohepatic circulation. Importantly, 5% of the bile acids are excreted and this accounts for the major loss of sterols from the body each day.

Studies in the last few years have demonstrated that nearly every step in the enterohepatic circulation is regulated by FXR (Figure 2). For example, cholesterol 7α-hydroxylase (CYP7A1), the rate-limiting enzyme in the classic pathway of bile acid synthesis [11], is repressed by bile acids returning to the liver from the intestine. It is now known that this repression results from multiple mechanisms. One mechanism involves FXR-dependent activation of the gene encoding the nuclear receptor SHP. Increased hepatic expression of SHP protein results in inactivation of liver receptor homolog 1 (LRH-1, NR5A2) as a result of interaction of SHP with LRH-1. Importantly, LRH-1 functions as a positive transcription factor that is necessary for *Cyp7a1* expression. Hence, CYP7A1 activity is repressed when SHP binds to and inactivates LRH-1 [24,25].

Activation of intestinal FXR by bile acids results in increased synthesis and secretion of murine fibroblast growth factor 15 (mouse FGF15/human FGF19). This growth factor has been shown to bind to the receptor, FGFR4, localized on the hepatocyte plasma membrane; the result is activation of the JNK pathway and repression of *Cyp7a1* expression [26]. Bile acids have also been shown to repress *Cyp7a1* via direct activation of the JNK pathway [27]. Thus, the regulation of *Cyp7a1* expression and the control of bile acid synthesis are complex and involve multiple levels of control, some of which involve FXR.

Once synthesized in the hepatocyte, bile acids are conjugated to taurine or glycine prior to their being pumped across the canalicular membrane by ABC transporters such as B*sep* and *Mdr2* (reviewed in [9,12]). The conjugating enzymes and the ABC transporters are regulated by FXR. Bile contains conjugated bile acids, phospholipids, cholesterol and relatively small amounts of proteins. Contraction of the gall bladder in response to food in the intestine expels the bile into the duodenum where it facilitates lipid digestion. Interestingly the subsequent relaxation and refilling of the gall bladder with bile is defective in *Fgf15$^{-/-}$* mice [28]. In these latter mice the gall bladder remains unfilled, consistent with a crucial role for *Fgf15* [28]. However, the role of FXR in this process remains to be established as *Fxr$^{-/-}$* mice appear to have normal sized gall bladders (unpublished data). It is possible that the levels of *Fgf15* protein in the *Fxr$^{-/-}$* mice are sufficient to allow normal or near normal relaxation and refilling of the gall bladder.

As stated above, 95% of the bile acids are reabsorbed from the intestinal lumen as part of the enterohepatic circulation. The apical sodium-dependent bile acid transporter (ASBT) involved in bile acid uptake into the enterocyte, the intestinal bile acid binding protein (IBABP) involved in transport across the enterocyte, and the organic solute transporter (OST)-α and OST-β that heterodimerize and pump bile acids out of the enterocyte and into the portal blood, are all FXR-target genes [12] (Figure 2).

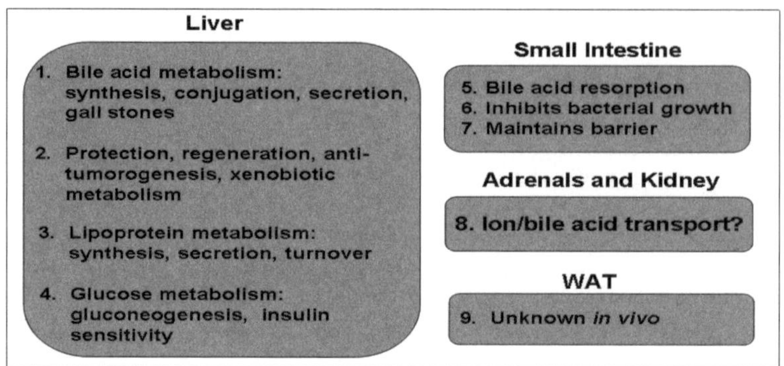

Figure 2. Multiple functions of FXR. High levels of FXR are expressed in the liver, small intestine, adrenal glands and kidney. FXR is also expressed at a low level in the white adipose tissue (WAT). The known functions of FXR in these tissues are shown.

One common imbalance in the enterohepatic circulation occurs when cholesterol begins to precipitate out in the gall bladder. Such a process occurs in millions of Americans and results in the formation of gall stones. Such cholesterol gall stones may become both large and painful. Gall stones are thought to form because of inappropriate solubilization of cholesterol by bile acids and phospholipids and/or from poor gall bladder motility. Recent studies demonstrated that gallstone-susceptible C57L mice had reduced gallstone formation following treatment of the mice with the FXR-agonist GW4064 [29]. It was proposed that such protection may result from increased transport of bile acids from the liver into bile as a result of FXR-dependent induction of the ABC transporters *Bsep* and *Mdr2* [29]. These data, together with evidence showing that FXR/FGF15 affects gall bladder filling suggests that FXR-agonists may be useful in regulating gall stone formation [28,29]. In summary, FXR is an important bile acid sensor that responds to changes in concentrations of bile acids by regulating many aspects of bile acid metabolism.

4. FXR and Plasma Cholesterol and Triglyceride Metabolism

In the early 1970s patients with gall stones were treated orally with bile acids in an attempt to slowly solubilize, and thus dissipate, the cholesterol-rich gall stones. This approach was based on the hypothesis that increasing the bile acid pool size would be beneficial. Indeed, this approach, although no longer in general use, had some clinical success in the treatment of gall stone disease. An interesting observation made at the time concerned the decline in levels of both plasma triglycerides and HDL in patients treated orally with bile acids (reviewed in [30]). The reason for these changes in plasma lipids was unknown. Interestingly, when the bile acid pool size was decreased, as a result either of treatment with bile acid sequestrants or following ileal surgery, plasma triglycerides and HDL levels increased (reviewed in [30]).

Studies with $Fxr^{-/-}$ mice, or following activation of FXR with bile acids or more specific FXR-agonists have revealed that these changes in plasma lipids, originally noted in humans, are a result of changes in gene expression that follow FXR-activation. These latter studies in rodents have shown that activation of hepatic FXR results in repression of SREBP-1C and that this repression likely accounts for the decline in fatty acid and triglyceride synthesis [31,32]. In addition, activation of FXR results in increased hepatic expression of the VLDL receptor and syndecan-1 that are involved in lipoprotein clearance, and in altered expression of proteins (ApoC-II, ApoC-III and ANGPTL3) that are known to modulate the activity of lipoprotein lipase (reviewed in [12]). The result of these changes in gene expression is a decrease in plasma triglycerides.

5. FXR and Glucose Metabolism

In addition to its role in regulating plasma lipids, recent studies have shown that FXR controls glucose homeostasis. Importantly, plasma glucose levels decline and insulin sensitivity increases when mice are treated with FXR-agonists, such as bile acids or GW4064, or when mice are infected with adenovirus that express a constitutively active form of FXR (FXR-VP16) [6,33,34]. Since adenoviral infection results in expression of FXR-VP16 only in the liver of the recipient mice, we have proposed that the hypoglycemic effects arise from activation of hepatic FXR [33]. The finding that the most profound hypoglycemic (and hypolipidemic) changes are observed following FXR-activation in diabetic mouse models (db/db, KK-A(y)) would appear to be significant. Whether such changes will prove to be of clinical importance remains to be determined.

FXR-activation in diabetic mice results in decreased hepatic phosphoenolpyruvate carboxykinase (PEPCK) and glucose-6-phosphatase (G6Pase) activity and to increased activity of glycogen synthase; the result is decreased gluconeogenesis and increased glycogen synthesis [33]. Activation of FXR in diabetic mice also improves insulin sensitivity in the liver [33]. Whether FXR-activation also affects insulin sensitivity in the muscle or white adipose tissue is unknown at this time.

Consistent with the hypoglycemic effects noted following FXR-activation, studies with $Fxr^{-/-}$ mice have shown that these mice exhibit i) reduced hepatic glycogen levels [35], ii) peripheral insulin resistance[6,34], iii) impaired glucose tolerance and insulin sensitivity [6,33,34] and iv) defective insulin signaling in the liver [34], and muscle [6,34]. It is not known whether the increased plasma free fatty acid levels of $Fxr^{-/-}$ mice contribute to these many phenotypes. Nonetheless, the current data suggest that FXR-activation may prove to be useful in the treatment of type-2 diabetes.

6. Additional Roles of FXR

The roles of FXR in atherosclerosis, in controlling bacterial growth in the intestine, in hepatic regeneration or hepatic tumor growth have all been recently described. Such topics are beyond the scope of this chapter. The interested readers are referred to the many reviews, some cited in the introduction to this chapter, for additional information.

7. Bile Acids and Gpbar

Recent studies have shown that administration of cholic acid-enriched diets to wild-type mice results in resistance to diet-induced obesity [18]. It has been proposed that this effect may be dependent upon the activation of a G-protein coupled receptor (Gpbar; TGR5) that is localized to the plasma membrane of numerous tissues including brown adipose tissue [18]. Activation of Gpbar *in vitro* by bile acids resulted in increased levels of cAMP in brown adipose tissue and increased expression of uncoupling proteins [18]. More recently it was reported that female, but not male, $Gpbar^{-/-}$ mice exhibit increased obesity following administration of a high-fat diet [36]. Whether this effect is dependent upon changes in plasma bile acids remains to be established.

Interestingly, $Fxr^{-/-}$ mice show small but significant increases in the plasma levels of bile acids [23] and exhibit resistance to diet-induced obesity (unpublished data). It will be of interest to determine whether such resistance to obesity is dependent upon bile acid activation of Gpbar or to some as yet unknown mechanism. In another study, particularly high levels of *Gpbar* mRNAs were detected in the gall bladder [37]. Based on the finding that $Gpbar^{-/-}$ mice were resistant to gall stone formation, a process that normally follows administration of a cholic-acid containing diet, the investigators concluded that Gpbar plays an important role in controlling gall stone formation [37]. Thus, bile acids function as critical agonists not only for the NRs FXR, PXR, CAR and VDR but also for a G-protein coupled receptor that affects gall stone formation and obesity. Clearly, the role of bile acids in controlling metabolic processes remains an area of particular interest, especially as the general population shows evidence of increasing levels of obesity and diabetes.

8. Conclusion

During the last 8 years our understanding of the function of bile acids has taken a radical new direction; it is now clear that bile acids function not only to facilitate lipid absorption but also are *bona fide* hormones that affect FXR and a number of other nuclear receptors, in addition to activating a G-protein coupled receptor, Gpbar. Such activations affect critical signaling pathways that in turn affect a variety of metabolic processes. Based on these findings, it seems possible that FXR-agonists may prove clinically useful to treat a number of metabolic disorders. However, the aim will be to identify synthetic modulators of FXR that provide sufficient specificity without regulating the many pathways affected by bile acids.

References

[1]   B.M. Forman, E. Goode, J. Chen *et al.* Identification of a nuclear receptor that is activated by farnesol metabolites. *Cell* **81** (1995) 687-693.

[2]   W. Seol, H.S. Choi, D.D. Moore. Isolation of proteins that interact specifically with the retinoid X receptor: two novel orphan receptors. *Mol. Endocrinol.* **9** (1995) 72-85.

[3]   W. Seol, H.S. Choi, D.D. Moore. An orphan nuclear hormone receptor that lacks a DNA binding domain and heterodimerizes with other receptors. *Science* **272** (1996) 1336-1339.

[4]   Y. Zhang, H.R. Kast-Woelbern, P.A. Edwards. Natural structural variants of the nuclear receptor farnesoid X receptor affect transcriptional activation. *J. Biol. Chem.* **278** (2003) 104-110.

[5]   R.M. Huber, K. Murphy, B. Miao *et al.* Generation of multiple farnesoid-X-receptor isoforms through the use of alternative promoters. *Gene* **290** (2002) 35-43.

[6]   B. Cariou, K. van Harmelen, D. Duran-Sandoval *et al.* The farnesoid X receptor modulates adiposity and peripheral insulin sensitivity in mice. *J. Biol. Chem.* **281** (2006) 11039-11049.

[7]   G. Rizzo, M. Disante, A. Mencarelli *et al.* The farnesoid X receptor promotes adipocyte differentiation and regulates adipose cell function in vivo. *Mol. Pharmacol.* **70** (2006) 1164-1173.

[8]   P.A. Edwards, H.R. Kast, A.M. Anisfeld. BAREing it all: the adoption of LXR and FXR and their roles in lipid homeostasis. *J. Lipid Res.* **43** (2002) 2-12.

[9]   N.Y. Kalaany and D.J. Mangelsdorf. LXRS and FXR: the yin and yang of cholesterol and fat metabolism. *Annu. Rev. Physiol.* **68** (2006) 159-191.

[10]   T. Claudel, E. Sturm, H. Duez *et al.* Bile acid-activated nuclear receptor FXR suppresses apolipoprotein A-I transcription via a negative FXR response element. *J. Clin. Invest.* **109** (2002) 961-971.

[11]   D.W. Russell. The enzymes, regulation, and genetics of bile acid synthesis. *Annu. Rev. Biochem.* **72** (2003) 137-174.

[12] F.Y. Lee, H. Lee, M.L. Hubbert *et al.* FXR, a multipurpose nuclear receptor. *Trends Biochem. Sci.* **31** (2006) 572-580.

[13] S.M. Houten, M. Watanabe, J. Auwerx. Endocrine functions of bile acids. *EMBO J.* **25** (2006) 1419-1425.

[14] M. Makishima, A.Y. Okamoto, J.J. Repa *et al.* Identification of a nuclear receptor for bile acids. *Science* **284** (1999) 1362-1365. Comment in: *Science* **284** (1999) 1285-1286.

[15] D.J. Parks, S.G. Blanchard, R.K. Bledsoe *et al.* Bile acids: natural ligands for an orphan nuclear receptor. *Science* **284** (1999) 1365-1368. Comment in: *Science* **284** (1999) 1285-1286.

[16] H. Wang, J. Chen, K. Hollister *et al.* Endogenous bile acids are ligands for the nuclear receptor FXR/BAR. *Mol. Cell* **3** (1999) 543-553.

[17] S. Wang, K. Lai, F.J. Moy *et al.* The nuclear hormone receptor farnesoid X receptor (FXR) is activated by androsterone. *Endocrinology* **147** (2006) 4025-4033.

[18] M. Watanabe, S.M. Houten, C. Mataki *et al.* Bile acids induce energy expenditure by promoting intracellular thyroid hormone activation. *Nature* **439** (2006) 484-489.

[19] P.R. Maloney, D.J. Parks, C.D. Haffner *et al.* Identification of a chemical tool for the orphan nuclear receptor FXR. *J. Med. Chem.* **43** (2000) 2971-2974.

[20] M. Downes, M.A. Verdecia, A.J. Roecker *et al.* A chemical, genetic, and structural analysis of the nuclear bile acid receptor FXR. *Mol. Cell* **11** (2003) 1079-1092. Comment in: *Mol. Cell* **11** (2003) 850-851.

[21] I. Dussault, R. Beard, M. Lin *et al.* Identification of gene-selective modulators of the bile acid receptor FXR. *J. Biol. Chem.* **278** (2003) 7027-7033.

[22] R. Pellicciari, S. Fiorucci, E. Camaioni *et al.* 6alpha-ethyl-chenodeoxycholic acid (6-ECDCA), a potent and selective FXR agonist endowed with anticholestatic activity. *J. Med. Chem.* **45** (2002) 3569-3572.

[23] C.J. Sinal, M. Tohkin, M. Miyata *et al.* Targeted disruption of the nuclear receptor FXR/BAR impairs bile acid and lipid homeostasis. *Cell* **102** (2000) 731-744.

[24] B. Goodwin, S.A. Jones, R.R. Price *et al.* A regulatory cascade of the nuclear receptors FXR, SHP-1, and LRH-1 represses bile acid biosynthesis. *Mol. Cell* **6** (2000) 517-526.

[25] T.T. Lu, M. Makishima, J.J. Repa *et al.* 2000. Molecular basis for feedback regulation of bile acid synthesis by nuclear receptors. *Mol. Cell* **6** (2000) 507-515.

[26] T. Inagaki, M. Choi, A. Moschetta *et al.* Fibroblast growth factor 15 functions as an enterohepatic signal to regulate bile acid homeostasis. *Cell Metab.* **2** (2005) 217-225.

[27] S. Gupta, R.T. Stravitz, P. Dent *et al.* Down-regulation of cholesterol 7alpha-hydroxylase (CYP7A1) gene expression by bile acids in primary rat hepatocytes is mediated by the c-Jun N-terminal kinase pathway. *J. Biol. Chem.* **276** (2001) 15816-15822.

[28] M. Choi, A. Moschetta, A.L. Bookout *et al.* Identification of a hormonal basis for gallbladder filling. *Nat. Med.* **12** (2006) 1253-1255.

[29] A. Moschetta, A.L. Bookout, D.J. Mangelsdorf. Prevention of cholesterol gallstone disease by FXR agonists in a mouse model. *Nat. Med.* **10** (2004) 1352-1358. Comment in: *Hepatology* **42** (2005) 218-221; *Nat. Med.* **10** (2004) 1301-1302.

[30] S. Modica and A. Moschetta. Nuclear bile acid receptor FXR as pharmacological target: are we there yet? *FEBS Lett.* **580** (2006) 5492-5499.

[31] M. Watanabe, S.M. Houten, L. Wang *et al.* Bile acids lower triglyceride levels via a pathway involving FXR, SHP, and SREBP-1c. *J. Clin. Invest.* **113** (2004) 1408-1418.

[32] Y. Zhang, L.W. Castellani, C.J. Sinal *et al.* Peroxisome proliferator-activated receptor-gamma coactivator 1alpha (PGC-1alpha) regulates triglyceride metabolism by activation of the nuclear receptor FXR. *Genes Dev.* **18** (2004) 157-169.

[33] Y. Zhang, F.Y. Lee, G. Barrera *et al.* Activation of the nuclear receptor FXR improves hyperglycemia and hyperlipidemia in diabetic mice. *Proc. Natl. Acad. Sci. U.S.A.* **103** (2006) 1006-1011.

[34] K. Ma, P.K. Saha, L. Chan *et al.* Farnesoid X receptor is essential for normal glucose homeostasis. *J. Clin. Invest.* **116** (2006) 1102-1109.

[35] B. Cariou, K. van Harmelen, D. Duran-Sandoval *et al.* Transient impairment of the adaptive response to fasting in FXR-deficient mice. *FEBS Lett.* **579** (2005) 4076-4080.

[36] T. Maruyama, K. Tanaka, J. Suzuki *et al.* Targeted disruption of G protein-coupled bile acid receptor 1 (Gpbar1/M-Bar) in mice. *J. Endocrinol.* **191** (2006) 197-205.

[37] G. Vassileva, A. Golovko, L. Markowitz *et al.* Targeted deletion of Gpbar1 protects mice from cholesterol gallstone formation. *Biochem. J.* **398** (2006) 423-430.

Nuclear Receptors as Molecular Targets for Cardiometabolic and Central Nervous System Diseases
J.L. Junien and B. Staels (Eds.)
IOS Press, 2008

51

The Role of PPARs in Human Prediabetes

Harald Staiger, Claus Thamer, Hans-Ulrich Häring
*Department of Internal Medicine, Division of Endocrinology, Diabetology, Angiology,
Nephrology, and Clinical Chemistry, Eberhard-Karls-University Tübingen, Otfried-Müller-
Strasse 10, 72076 Tübingen, Germany*

Abstract. PPARs are important regulators of lipid and glucose metabolism. Clinical
trials assessing the efficacy of fibrates and thiazolidinediones in the treatment of
dyslipidemia and insulin resistance and recent genetic studies evaluating the impact
of genetic variation in genes encoding PPARs on prediabetic phenotypes, such as
insulin resistance, β-cell dysfunction, subclinical inflammation, and ectopic lipid
deposition, revealed the importance of these nuclear hormone receptors in human
metabolic disease. These findings as well as novel aspects of the role of PPARs in
human metabolism are summarized herein.

Keywords. Single nucleotide polymorphism, insulin sensitivity, insulin secretion,
dyslipidemia, inflammation, metabolic disease

1. Cellular and Metabolic Functions of PPARs

The nuclear hormone receptors of the peroxisome proliferator-activated receptor (PPAR)
family are important ligand-dependent transcriptional regulators of metabolic pathways.
Upon ligand-binding, PPARs adopt an active conformation and heterodimerize with
Retinoid X Receptors (RXR). These complexes bind to specific DNA sequences within
gene enhancer structures, so-called PPAR response elements (PPREs). Via recruitment of
co-activator proteins, PPAR-RXR complexes transactivate target gene promoters. Three
PPAR isoforms encoded by distinct genes are present in the human genome: PPARα
(NR1C1; gene: *PPARA*; chromosome 22q12-q13.1)
http://www.ncbi.nlm.nih.gov/entrez/viewer.fcgi?val=L02932, PPARγ (NR1C3; gene:
PPARG; chromosome 3p25), and PPARδ (NR1C2; gene: *PPARD*; chromosome 6p21.2).

PPARα is nearly ubiquitously expressed with highest expression levels in tissues of
high fatty acid oxidative capacity, such as brown adipose tissue, liver, kidney, heart and
skeletal muscle. Natural ligands of PPARα are long-chain (≥C18) unsaturated fatty acids
and arachidonic acid derivatives, such as 8(S)-hydroxyeicosatetraenoic acid and leukotriene
B4 [1], oxidized phospholipids derived from oxidized-low-density lipoproteins (LDL) [2],
and oleylethanolamide [3]. Among the pharmacological PPARα agonists, the fibrate class
of drugs, including fenofibrate, bezafibrate, and gemfibrozil, achieved clinical relevance in
the treatment of hypertriglyceridemia (for review, see [4]). The metabolic function of
PPARα was most extensively assessed in the liver where this receptor revealed an
important role in the cellular response to fasting [5]. Upon activation in the fasting state,
PPARα mediates fatty acid oxidation, gluconeogenesis, ketone body and high-density
lipoprotein (HDL) formation [5-8]. Moreover, PPARα activation not only reduces
circulating triglycerides and elevates plasma HDL levels [4], but also counteracts ectopic

lipid deposition in liver and muscle, obesity, and insulin resistance [9-11]. Consistent with its physiological effects, PPARα activation was shown to induce genes involved in hepatocellular fatty acid uptake, intracellular fatty acid binding, mitochondrial, peroxisomal, and microsomal fatty acid oxidation, and lipoprotein metabolism (for review, see [12]).

PPARγ exists in two isoforms, PPARγ1 and PPARγ2, which arise from alternative promoter usage and differ at their NH_2-terminus. PPARγ2 is predominantly expressed in adipose tissue, whereas PPARγ1 displays a broader distribution with detectable levels in adipose tissue, gut, brain, vasculature, immune cells, retina, kidney, liver, and skeletal muscle. Both isoforms are similarly activated and functionally undistinguishable. Among the naturally occuring ligands, 15-deoxy-$\Delta^{12,14}$-prostaglandin J2 [13] and the prostaglandins H1 and H2 [13,14] represent the most potent PPARγ activators. The thiazolidinediones (TZDs) rosiglitazone and pioglitazone, which are clinically used as insulin sensitizers in the treatment of type-2 diabetes, act as high-affinity pharmacological PPARγ agonists (for review, see [15]). PPARγ represents a master regulator of adipogenesis and lipogenesis, and its activation drives the expression of genes involved in adipocellular fatty acid uptake, intracellular fatty acid binding, and fatty acid synthesis, and modulates the expression of adipocyte-derived hormones (adipokines) [16,17]. The effect of PPARγ activation on insulin sensitivity is far from being molecularly clarified, but is currently suggested to be due to *de novo* formation of small insulin-sensitive adipocytes at the expense of hypertrophic insulin-resistant adipocytes [18,19] and induction of adiponectin, an insulin-sensitizing adipokine [15,20,21].

PPARδ is considered to be ubiquitously expressed and is activated by long-chain (≥C18) unsaturated fatty acids. GW501516 and L165041 represent PPARδ-selective synthetic ligands available for laboratory use only [22,23], and no pharmacological PPARδ agonists are currently in clinical use. PPARδ's cellular functions are up to now best studied in skeletal muscle where PPARδ activation induces the expression of structural genes encoding type I myofibre components and genes involved in fatty acid oxidation, mitochondrial respiration, and adaptive thermogenesis [24-27]. Physiologically, PPARδ activation was shown to promote a fibre type switch from white glycolytic to red oxidative myofibres, to stimulate mitochondriogenesis, and to counteract obesity and insulin resistance [24,25,28,29].

2. The Role of PPARs in Human Metabolic Disease: Results from Clinical Studies

Several clinical trials, such as the Helsinki Heart Study, the Veterans Affairs High-density lipoprotein Intervention Trial (VA-HIT), the Diabetes Atherosclerosis Intervention Study (DAIS), the Bezafibrate Infarction Prevention (BIP) trial, and the Fenofibrate Intervention and Event Lowering in Diabetes (FIELD) study, were conducted to test fibrates for the treatment of hypertriglyceridemia and low HDL levels in obese, insulin-resistant, and type-2 diabetic patients, and most of these studies revealed a good efficacy of the PPARα agonists in the treatment of these pro-atherogenic blood parameters (for review, see [30]). Thus, the clinical evidences for metabolic effects of PPARα activation clearly confirm the results derived from *in vitro* and mouse studies. As to the end point cardiovascular disease however, the results of the trials are inconsistent [31]. Therefore, a meta-analysis was recently performed to evaluate the role of fibrates in the prevention of cardiovascular events and revealed that long-term use of fibrates significantly reduces the occurrence of non-fatal myocardial infarction, but has no significant effect on other adverse cardiovascular outcomes [32].

With regard to TZDs, a plethora of clinical studies including large clinical trials, such as A Diabetes Outcome Progression Trial (ADOPT) and the Diabetes REduction Assessment with ramipril and rosiglitazone Medication (DREAM), consistently document the insulin-sensitizing and anti-hyperglycemic effects of the PPARγ agonists in prediabetic and type-2 diabetic patients (for review, see [33]). An important aspect of these TZD actions is elevation of plasma adiponectin levels [21,34-36] which closely reflects the laboratory findings on the role of PPARγ in the regulation of the adiponectin gene. Furthermore, TZDs are suggested to improve β-cell survival and function (reviewed in [37]) and to ameliorate several risk factors for cardiovascular disease, as derived from the PROspective pioglitAzone Clinical Trial In macroVascular Events (PROactive) trial [38] and the Carotid Intima-media Thickness in Atherosclerosis using Pioglitazone (CHICAGO) trial [39]. However, one major drawback for a more common use of TZDs in practice is the frequently reported increase in body weight that clearly represents a class effect of TZDs [40] and is in line with the well-documented adipogenic and lipogenic functions of PPARγ.

No clinical trail on the role of PPARδ in metabolic disease is reported due to the lack of PPARδ agonists available for clinical use.

3. Impact of the *PPARG* Gene on Prediabetic Phenotypes

It is generally agreed that obesity, type-2 diabetes, and the metabolic syndrome are metabolic disorders caused by environmental factors (e.g. high-caloric diets), behaviour (sedentary lifestyle), and a polygenic background. To identify the responsible genes and gene variants, candidate gene approaches, positional cloning efforts, and, very recently, genome-wide association studies were undertaken. Initiated by the plenty of metabolic *in vitro* and *in vivo* data on PPARγ, the *PPARG* gene was among the first candidate genes for obesity and type-2 diabetes. Two *PPARG* single nucleotide polymorphisms (SNPs) common in Caucasians (minor allele frequency, MAF >0.1) were identified in the late 1990s: a missense mutation leading to a Pro12Ala amino-acid exchange in the PPARγ2 protein (dbSNP identifier: rs1801282) and a silent +1431C→T mutation in the coding exon 6 (dbSNP identifier: rs3856806) [41] which are in ~70 % linkage disequilibrium. Cross-sectional studies revealed association of both SNPs' minor alleles with higher body mass index (BMI) [42-44] and increased insulin sensitivity, particularly in obese subjects [45-47]. Interestingly, the Ala allele of the Pro12Ala mutation, which displays lower transcriptional activity [48], was demonstrated to associate with lower plasma free fatty acid levels [49] due to enhanced insulin sensitivity of adipose tissue lipolysis [50-52], to associate with elevated hepatic insulin clearance [49], to allow better suppression of lipid oxidation [53], and to confer increased susceptibility towards the negative effects of fatty acids on the 2nd-phase of glucose-stimulated insulin secretion and on arginine-stimulated insulin secretion [54].

Even though cross-sectional studies turned out to be appropriate to detect prominent metabolic effects of genetic variants, small but yet clinically meaningful SNP effects can remain undetected. Intervention studies represent a more suitable approach to capture even small SNP effects on intervention-induced changes in metabolic traits. The TUebingen Lifestyle Intervention Program (TULIP) is an ongoing controlled dietary and exercise intervention study designed to unravel the genetic causes of prediabetic phenotypes, such as insulin resistance, β-cell dysfunction, subclinical inflammation, and ectopic lipid deposition, in thoroughly phenotyped subjects at an increased risk for type-2 diabetes (risk factors: overweight, family history of diabetes, history of gestational diabetes). The success of this lifestyle intervention was recently documented [55-58]. In this cohort, we observed that carriers of the Ala allele of *PPARG* Pro12Ala display significantly more pronounced intervention-induced decrements in plasma C-reactive protein levels and substantially higher increments in flow-mediated vasodilation, a measure of endothelial function (Figure 1 and [59]). These findings support the suggestion that the Ala allele may also confer a reduced risk of atherosclerosis to the SNP carriers [60,61].

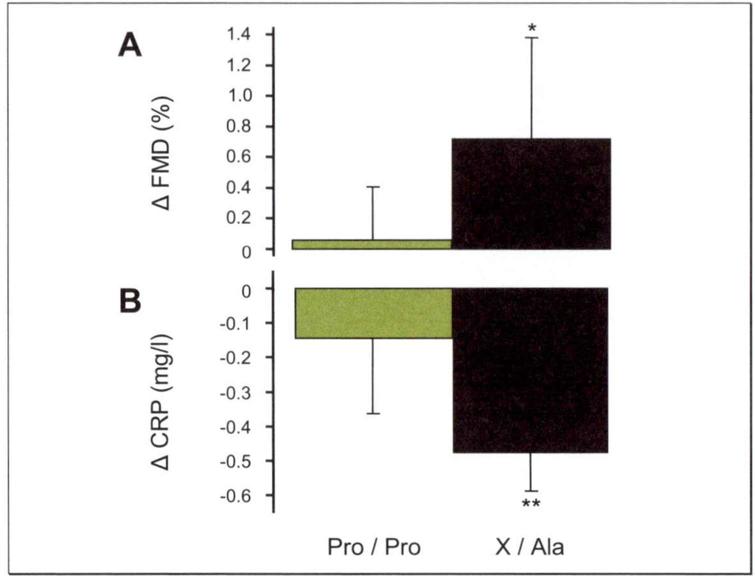

Figure 1. Changes in flow-mediated vasodilation (FMD, A) and plasma C-reactive protein levels (CRP, B) during lifestyle intervention in individuals carrying the *PPARG* Pro/Pro and X/Ala genotype (from [59]).

Finally, the importance of *PPARG* as a type-2 diabetes candidate gene was evidenced in case-control studies (for meta-analysis, see [62]) as well as in prospective studies [63,64] and was confirmed in recent genome-wide association studies [65-67].

4. Impact of the *PPARD* Gene on Prediabetic Phenotypes

The *PPARD* gene joined the field of metabolic research in 2003, when it was reported that the minor allele of the common SNP +294T→C in the 5'-untranslated region (dbSNP identifier: rs2016520) associates with higher plasma LDL as well as lower HDL cholesterol levels [68-70] and, in addition, with an increased risk of coronary heart disease [71]. More recently, this SNP was found to confer a lower BMI to the SNP carriers [72]. Furthermore, two common SNPs located within a linkage block encompassing exons 7-11, namely the silent mutation rs2076167 in exon 7 and SNP rs1053049 in the 3'-untranslated region, as well as the less frequent intronic SNP rs6902123 (MAF ~0.07) were identified that were associated with significantly increased whole-body glucose uptake due to elevated skeletal muscle, but not adipose tissue, glucose uptake [73]. In the TULIP study, carriers of the minor G allele of another SNP, i.e. the intronic SNP rs2267668, which is in close linkage disequilibrium with SNP +294T→C, revealed lower intervention-induced increments in insulin sensitivity and aerobic physical fitness resulting from reduced myocellular mitochondrial function (Figure 2 and [56]). The latter findings are in keeping with results from the HEalth, RIsk factors, exercise Training And GEnetics (HERITAGE) family study demonstrating an association of SNP +294T→C with reduced physical performance during endurance training [74].

Even though the aforementioned reports confirm PPARδ's importance for human muscle metabolism, the metabolic role of PPARδ is probably not limited to skeletal muscle. More recent data from the TULIP study provide evidence that SNP rs1053049 in the 3'-untranslated region and the intronic SNP rs6902123 impair not only the intervention-induced increment in muscle volume but also the intervention-induced decrements in adiposity and hepatic lipid content (C. Thamer *et al, J. Clin. Endocrinol. Metab.*, manuscript submitted for publication). These observations point to PPARδ-dependent metabolic and/or humoral cross-talk pathways linking skeletal muscle, presumably the primary site of PPARδ action, with adipose tissue and liver.

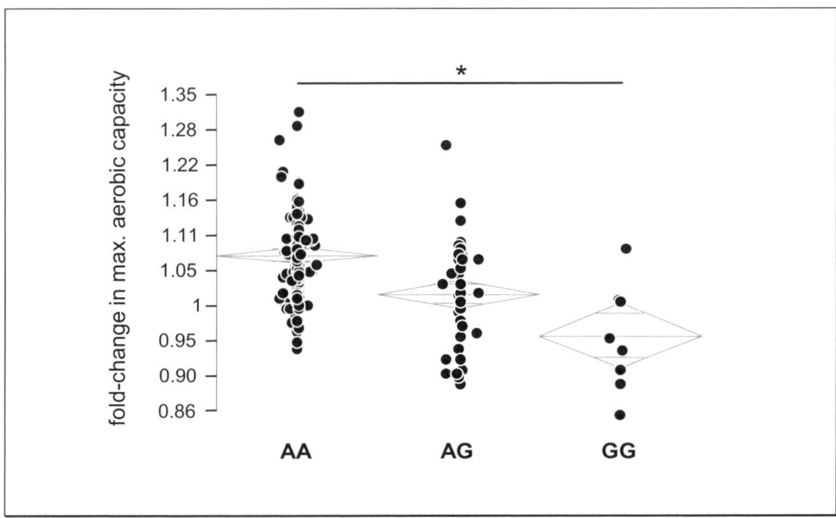

Figure 2. Changes in maximum aerobic capacity during lifestyle intervention in individuals carrying the *PPARD* SNP rs2267668 (from [56]).

Up to now, only in one cohort, i.e. the Study to Prevent Non-Insulin-Dependent Diabetes Mellitus (STOP-NIDDM), the question was addressed whether genetic variation within the *PPARD* gene contributes to the risk of type-2 diabetes, and SNP rs6902123 was found to increase the risk of type-2 diabetes 2.7-fold in women, but not in men [75].

5. Novel Aspects of PPARδ Action: Mediation of Humoral Cross-talk between Muscle and Adipose Tissue

The supposed PPARδ-dependent cross-talk mechanisms are thought to include altered substrate fluxes due to PPARδ's potent lipid-burning properties in muscle and/or altered expression of muscle-derived secretory factors (myokines). Myokines represent a rather novel field of research initiated by the characterization of muscle-derived interleukin 6 as a systemically acting exercise factor (for review, see [76]). Our group recently identified *ANGPTL4* as the gene most responsive to non-esterified long-chain fatty acids in human skeletal muscle cells, and this gene induction was found to be mediated by PPARδ activation (H. Staiger *et al, Diabetes*, manuscript submitted for publication).

ANGPTL4 encodes angiopoietin-like protein 4 (ANGPTL4), a secreted protein which was previously shown in mice to be predominantly produced by adipose tissue and liver and to affect lipid metabolism in two ways: (i) via inhibition of lipoprotein lipase, ANGPTL4 inhibits the clearance of very-low-density lipoproteins (VLDL) and chylomicrons thus provoking hypertriglyceridemia [77-81]; and (ii) via induction of adipose triglyceride lipase, ANGPTL4 stimulates adipose tissue lipolysis [82] and elevates plasma glycerol and non-esterified fatty acid levels [77,82]. Besides hyperlipidemia, ANGPTL4 promotes adipose tissue weight loss and hepatic steatosis [79,82]. In humans, we demonstrated, in a translational setting, that muscle cell *ANGPTL4* expression *in vitro* reflects adipose tissue lipolysis of the donors *in vivo*, and this finding prompted us to establish the hypothesis that PPARδ activation in skeletal muscle via ANGPTL4 production constitutes a humoral muscle - adipose tissue axis (Figure 3 and H. Staiger *et al*, *Diabetes*, manuscript submitted for publication).

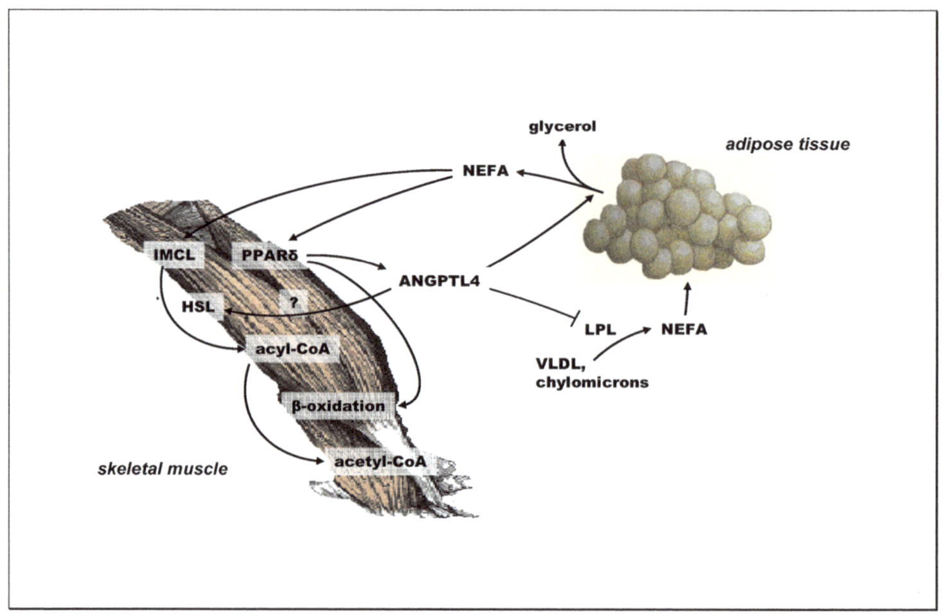

Figure 3. Hypothetical role of PPARδ-mediated muscle ANGPTL4 secretion. In states of increased muscle PPARδ activity, such as fasting and exercise, skeletal muscle secretes ANGPTL4. Simultaneously, muscular fatty acid oxidation is increased by PPARδ-dependent induction of β-oxidative enzymes. Via the circulation, ANGPTL4 enhances adipose tissue lipolysis and thus ensures ongoing fuel supply of the stressed muscle. Together with ANGPTL4's suggested inhibitory effect on lipoprotein lipase, this mechanism is expected to provoke loss of adipose tissue mass (from H. Staiger *et al*, *Diabetes*, submitted).

6. Concluding Remarks

There is currently no doubt that PPARs represent important regulators of human lipid and glucose metabolism. In particular, it is the *PPARG* gene that turned out to be a relevant type-2 diabetes candidate gene. The recent findings on the metabolic functions of PPARδ open new and promising directions in the field of hormone, diabetes, and atherosclerosis research. However, PPARs are subject to a very complex molecular regulation by ligand-binding, heterodimerization with RXR isoforms, and recruitment of diverse co-repressor and co-activator proteins. Therefore, much is still to be learned about the molecular biology and physiology of PPARs in order to estimate all their functions in human metabolism and beyond and in order to develop safe and highly specific pharmacological drugs for the therapy of metabolic diseases.

References

[1] Q. Lin, S.E. Ruuska, N.S. Shaw *et al.* Ligand selectivity of the peroxisome proliferator-activated receptor alpha. *Biochemistry* **38** (1999) 185-190.

[2] P. Delerive, C. Furman, E. Teissier *et al.* Oxidized phospholipids activate PPARalpha in a phospholipase A2-dependent manner. *FEBS Lett.* **471** (2000) 34-38.

[3] J. Fu, S. Gaetani, F. Oveisi *et al.* Oleylethanolamide regulates feeding and body weight through activation of the nuclear receptor PPAR-alpha. *Nature* **425** (2003) 90-93.

[4] J.C. Fruchart and P. Duriez. Mode of action of fibrates in the regulation of triglyceride and HDL-cholesterol metabolism. *Drugs Today (Barc).* **42** (2006) 39-64.

[5] S. Kersten, J. Seydoux, J.M. Peters *et al.* Peroxisome proliferator-activated receptor alpha mediates the adaptive response to fasting. *J. Clin. Invest.* **103** (1999) 1489-1498.

[6] T.C. Leone, C.J. Weinheimer, D.P. Kelly. A critical role for the peroxisome proliferator-activated receptor alpha (PPARalpha) in the cellular fasting response: the PPARalpha-null mouse as a model of fatty acid oxidation disorders. *Proc. Natl. Acad. Sci. U.S.A.* **96** (1999) 7473-7478.

[7] J.M. Peters, N. Hennuyer, B. Staels *et al.* Alterations in lipoprotein metabolism in peroxisome proliferator-activated receptor alpha-deficient mice. *J. Biol. Chem.* **272** (1997) 27307-27312.

[8] T. Aoyama, J.M. Peters, N. Iritani *et al.* Altered constitutive expression of fatty acid-metabolizing enzymes in mice lacking the peroxisome proliferator-activated receptor alpha (PPARalpha). *J. Biol. Chem.* **273** (1998) 5678-5684.

[9] C.J. Chou, M. Haluzik, C. Gregory *et al.* WY14,643, a peroxisome proliferator-activated receptor alpha (PPARalpha) agonist, improves hepatic and muscle steatosis and reverses insulin resistance in lipoatrophic A-ZIP/F-1 mice. *J. Biol. Chem.* **277** (2002) 24484-24489.

[10] M. Guerre-Millo, P. Gervois, E. Raspé *et al.* Peroxisome proliferator-activated receptor alpha activators improve insulin sensitivity and reduce adiposity. *J. Biol. Chem.* **275** (2000) 16638-16642.

[11] H. Kim, M. Haluzik, Z. Asghar *et al.* Peroxisome proliferator-activated receptor-alpha agonist treatment in a transgenic model of type 2 diabetes reverses the lipotoxic state and improves glucose homeostasis. *Diabetes* **52** (2003) 1770-1778.

[12] S. Mandard, M. Müller, S. Kersten. Peroxisome proliferator-activated receptor alpha target genes. *Cell Mol. Life Sci.* **61** (2004) 393-416.

[13] B.M. Forman, P. Tontonoz, J. Chen *et al.* 15-Deoxy-delta 12,14-prostaglandin J2 is a ligand for the adipocyte determination factor PPAR gamma. *Cell* **83** (1995) 803-812.

[14] G. Ferry, V. Bruneau, P. Beauverger *et al.* Binding of prostaglandins to human PPARgamma: tool assessment and new natural ligands. *Eur. J. Pharmacol.* **417** (2001) 77-89.

[15] M. Stumvoll and H.U. Häring. Glitazones: clinical effects and molecular mechanisms. *Ann. Med.* **34** (2002) 217-224.

[16] B.M. Spiegelman. Peroxisome proliferator-activated receptor gamma: A key regulator of adipogenesis and systemic insulin sensitivity. *Eur. J. Med. Res.* **2** (1997) 457-464.

[17] B.B. Lowell. PPARgamma: an essential regulator of adipogenesis and modulator of fat cell function. *Cell* **99** (1999) 239-242.

[18] A. Okuno, H. Tamemoto, K. Tobe *et al.* Troglitazone increases the number of small adipocytes without the change of white adipose tissue mass in obese Zucker rats. *J. Clin. Invest.* **101** (1998) 1354-1361.

[19] H. Minoura, S. Takeshita, C. Kimura *et al.* Mechanism by which a novel non-thiazolidinedione peroxisome proliferator-activated receptor gamma agonist, FK614, ameliorates insulin resistance in Zucker fatty rats. *Diabetes Obes. Metab.* **9** (2007) 369-378.

[20] N. Maeda, M. Takahashi, T. Funahashi *et al.* PPARgamma ligands increase expression and plasma concentrations of adiponectin, an adipose-derived protein. *Diabetes* **50** (2001) 2094-2099.

[21] J.G. Yu, S. Javorschi, A.L. Hevener *et al.* The effect of thiazolidinediones on plasma adiponectin levels in normal, obese, and type 2 diabetic subjects. *Diabetes* **51** (2002) 2968-2974.

[22] M.L. Sznaidman, C.D. Haffner, P.R. Maloney *et al.* Novel selective small molecule agonists for peroxisome proliferator-activated receptor delta (PPARdelta)--synthesis and biological activity. *Bioorg. Med. Chem. Lett.* **13** (2003) 1517-1521.

[23] P. Pelton. GW-501516 GlaxoSmithKline/Ligand. *Curr. Opin. Investig. Drugs* **7** (2006) 360-370.

[24]	Y.X. Wang, C.L. Zhang, R.T. Yu *et al.* Regulation of muscle fiber type and running endurance by PPARdelta. *PLoS Biol.* **2** (2004) e294. Erratum in: *PLoS Biol.* **3** (2005) e61.

[25]	Y.X. Wang, C.H. Lee, S. Tiep *et al.* Peroxisome-proliferator-activated receptor delta activates fat metabolism to prevent obesity. *Cell* **113** (2003) 159-170.

[26]	U. Dressel, T.L. Allen, J.B. Pippal *et al.* The peroxisome proliferator-activated receptor beta/delta agonist, GW501516, regulates the expression of genes involved in lipid catabolism and energy uncoupling in skeletal muscle cells. *Mol. Endocrinol.* **17** (2003) 2477-2493.

[27]	E. Chevillotte, J. Rieusset, M. Roques *et al.* The regulation of uncoupling protein-2 gene expression by omega-6 polyunsaturated fatty acids in human skeletal muscle cells involves multiple pathways, including the nuclear receptor peroxisome proliferator-activated receptor beta. *J. Biol. Chem.* **276** (2001) 10853-10860.

[28]	T. Tanaka, J. Yamamoto, S. Iwasaki *et al.* Activation of peroxisome proliferator-activated receptor delta induces fatty acid beta-oxidation in skeletal muscle and attenuates metabolic syndrome. *Proc. Natl. Acad. Sci. U.S.A.* **100** (2003) 15924-15929.

[29]	C.H. Lee, P. Olson, A. Hevener *et al.* PPARdelta regulates glucose metabolism and insulin sensitivity. *Proc. Natl. Acad. Sci. U.S.A.* **103** (2006) 3444-3449.

[30]	S. Fazio and M.F. Linton. The role of fibrates in managing hyperlipidemia: mechanisms of action and clinical efficacy. *Curr. Atheroscler. Rep.* **6** (2004) 148-157.

[31]	J.M. Backes, C.A. Gibson, J.F. Ruisinger *et al.* Fibrates: what have we learned in the past 40 years? *Pharmacotherapy* **27** (2007) 412-424.

[32]	S.A. Saha, L.G. Kizhakepunnur, A. Bahekar *et al.* The role of fibrates in the prevention of cardiovascular disease--a pooled meta-analysis of long-term randomized placebo-controlled clinical trials. *Am. Heart J.* **154** (2007) 943-953.

[33]	R.B. Goldberg. The new clinical trials with thiazolidinediones--DREAM, ADOPT, and CHICAGO: promises fulfilled? *Curr. Opin. Lipidol.* **18** (2007) 435-442.

[34]	S.A. Phillips, T.P. Ciaraldi, A.P. Kong *et al.* Modulation of circulating and adipose tissue adiponectin levels by antidiabetic therapy. *Diabetes* **52** (2003) 667-674.

[35]	J. Tonelli, W. Li, P. Kishore *et al.* Mechanisms of early insulin-sensitizing effects of thiazolidinediones in type 2 diabetes. *Diabetes* **53** (2004) 1621-1629. Erratum in: *Diabetes* **54** (2005) 587.

[36]	Y. Miyazaki, A. Mahankali, E. Wajcberg *et al.* Effect of pioglitazone on circulating adipocytokine levels and insulin sensitivity in type 2 diabetic patients. *J. Clin. Endocrinol. Metab.* **89** (2004) 4312-4319.

[37]	I.W. Campbell and S. Mariz. Beta-cell preservation with thiazolidinediones. *Diabetes Res. Clin. Pract.* **76** (2007) 163-176.

[38]	J.A. Dormandy, B. Charbonnel, D.J. Eckland *et al.* Secondary prevention of macrovascular events in patients with type 2 diabetes in the PROactive Study (PROspective pioglitAzone Clinical Trial In macroVascular Events): a randomised controlled trial. *Lancet* **366** (2005) 1279-1289.

[39]	T. Mazzone, P.M. Meyer, S.B. Feinstein *et al.* Effect of pioglitazone compared with glimepiride on carotid intima-media thickness in type 2 diabetes: a randomized trial. *JAMA* **296** (2006) 2572-2581.

[40]	J. Wilding. Thiazolidinediones, insulin resistance and obesity: Finding a balance. *Int. J. Clin. Pract.* **60** (2006) 1272-1280.

[41]	C.J. Yen, B.A. Beamer, C. Negri *et al.* Molecular scanning of the human peroxisome proliferator activated receptor gamma (hPPAR gamma) gene in diabetic Caucasians: identification of a Pro12Ala PPAR gamma 2 missense mutation. *Biochem. Biophys. Res. Commun.* **241** (1997) 270-274.

[42]	B.A. Beamer, C.J. Yen, R.E. Andersen *et al.* Association of the Pro12Ala variant in the peroxisome proliferator-activated receptor-gamma2 gene with obesity in two Caucasian populations. *Diabetes* **47** (1998) 1806-1808.

[43]	A. Meirhaeghe, L. Fajas, N. Helbecque *et al.* A genetic polymorphism of the peroxisome proliferator-activated receptor gamma gene influences plasma leptin levels in obese humans. *Hum. Mol. Genet.* **7** (1998) 435-440.

[44]	R. Valve, K. Sivenius, R. Miettinen *et al.* Two polymorphisms in the peroxisome proliferator-activated receptor-gamma gene are associated with severe overweight among obese women. *J. Clin. Endocrinol. Metab.* **84** (1999) 3708-3712.

[45]	M. Koch, K. Rett, E. Maerker *et al.* The PPARgamma2 amino acid polymorphism Pro 12 Ala is prevalent in offspring of Type II diabetic patients and is associated to increased insulin sensitivity in a subgroup of obese subjects. *Diabetologia* **42** (1999) 758-762.

[46]	K. Hara, T. Okada, K. Tobe *et al.* The Pro12Ala polymorphism in PPAR gamma2 may confer resistance to type 2 diabetes. *Biochem. Biophys. Res. Commun.* **271** (2000) 212-216.

[47]	M. Stumvoll, N. Stefan, A. Fritsche *et al.* Interaction effect between common polymorphisms in PPARgamma2 (Pro12Ala) and insulin receptor substrate 1 (Gly972Arg) on insulin sensitivity. *J. Mol. Med.* **80** (2002) 33-38.

[48] S.S. Deeb, L. Fajas, M. Nemoto *et al.* A Pro12Ala substitution in PPARgamma2 associated with decreased receptor activity, lower body mass index and improved insulin sensitivity. *Nat. Genet.* **20** (1998) 284-287.

[49] O. Tschritter, A. Fritsche, N. Stefan *et al.* Increased insulin clearance in peroxisome proliferator-activated receptor gamma2 Pro12Ala. *Metabolism* **52** (2003) 778-783.

[50] S. Jacob, M. Stumvoll, R. Becker *et al.* The PPARgamma2 polymorphism pro12Ala is associated with better insulin sensitivity in the offspring of type 2 diabetic patients. *Horm. Metab. Res.* **32** (2000) 413-416.

[51] M. Stumvoll, H.G. Wahl, K. Löblein *et al.* Pro12Ala polymorphism in the peroxisome proliferator-activated receptor-gamma2 gene is associated with increased antilipolytic insulin sensitivity. *Diabetes* **50** (2001) 876-881.

[52] M. Stumvoll and H. Häring. Reduced lipolysis as possible cause for greater weight gain in subjects with the Pro12Ala polymorphism in PPARgamma2? *Diabetologia* **45** (2002) 152-153.

[53] C. Thamer, M. Haap, A. Volk *et al.* Evidence for greater oxidative substrate flexibility in male carriers of the Pro 12 Ala polymorphism in PPARgamma2. *Horm. Metab. Res.* **34** (2002) 132-136.

[54] N. Stefan, A. Fritsche, H. Häring *et al.* Effect of experimental elevation of free fatty acids on insulin secretion and insulin sensitivity in healthy carriers of the Pro12Ala polymorphism of the peroxisome proliferator--activated receptor-gamma2 gene. *Diabetes* **50** (2001) 1143-1148.

[55] S. Schäfer, K. Kantartzis, J. Machann *et al.* Lifestyle intervention in individuals with normal versus impaired glucose tolerance. *Eur. J. Clin. Invest.* **37** (2007) 535-543.

[56] N. Stefan, C. Thamer, H. Staiger *et al.* Genetic variations in PPARD and PPARGC1A determine mitochondrial function and change in aerobic physical fitness and insulin sensitivity during lifestyle intervention. *J. Clin. Endocrinol. Metab.* **92** (2007) 1827-1833.

[57] C. Thamer, J. Machann, N. Stefan *et al.* High visceral fat mass and high liver fat are associated with resistance to lifestyle intervention. *Obesity (Silver Spring)* **15** (2007) 531-538.

[58] P. Weyrich, N. Stefan, H.U. Häring *et al.* Effect of genotype on success of lifestyle intervention in subjects at risk for type 2 diabetes. *J. Mol. Med.* **85** (2007) 107-117.

[59] K. Rittig, C. Thamer, F. Machicao *et al.* The Pro12Ala polymorphism in PPARG2 increases the effectiveness of primary prevention of cardiovascular disease by a lifestyle intervention. *Diabetologia* **50** (2007) 1345-1347.

[60] E. Iwata, I. Yamamoto, T. Motomura *et al.* The association of Pro12Ala polymorphism in PPARgamma2 with lower carotid artery IMT in Japanese. *Diabetes Res. Clin. Pract.* **62** (2003) 55-59.

[61] B.C. Lee, H.J. Lee, J.H. Chung. Peroxisome proliferator-activated receptor-gamma2 Pro12Ala polymorphism is associated with reduced risk for ischemic stroke with type 2 diabetes. *Neurosci. Lett.* **410** (2006) 141-145.

[62] D. Altshuler, J.N. Hirschhorn, M. Klannemark *et al.* The common PPARgamma Pro12Ala polymorphism is associated with decreased risk of type 2 diabetes. *Nat. Genet.* **26** (2000) 76-80.

[63] A. Memisoglu, F.B. Hu, S.E. Hankinson *et al.* Prospective study of the association between the proline to alanine codon 12 polymorphism in the PPARgamma gene and type 2 diabetes. *Diabetes Care* **26** (2003) 2915-2917.

[64] R. Jaziri, S. Lobbens, R. Aubert *et al.* The PPARG Pro12Ala polymorphism is associated with a decreased risk of developing hyperglycemia over 6 years and combines with the effect of the APM1 G-11391A single nucleotide polymorphism: the Data From an Epidemiological Study on the Insulin Resistance Syndrome (DESIR) study. *Diabetes* **55** (2006) 1157-1162.

[65] R. Saxena, B.F. Voight, V. Lyssenko *et al.* Genome-wide association analysis identifies loci for type 2 diabetes and triglyceride levels. *Science* **316** (2007) 1331-1336.

[66] E. Zeggini, M.N. Weedon, C.M. Lindgren *et al.* Replication of genome-wide association signals in UK samples reveals risk loci for type 2 diabetes. *Science* **316** (2007) 1336-1341. Erratum in: *Science* **317** (2007) 1035-1036.

[67] L.J. Scott, K.L. Mohlke, L.L. Bonnycastle *et al.* A genome-wide association study of type 2 diabetes in Finns detects multiple susceptibility variants. *Science* **316** (2007) 1341-1345.

[68] J. Skogsberg, K. Kannisto, T.N. Cassel *et al.* Evidence that peroxisome proliferator-activated receptor delta influences cholesterol metabolism in men. *Arterioscler. Thromb. Vasc. Biol.* **23** (2003) 637-643.

[69] J. Skogsberg, A.D. McMahon, F. Karpe *et al.* Peroxisome proliferator activated receptor delta genotype in relation to cardiovascular risk factors and risk of coronary heart disease in hypercholesterolaemic men. *J. Intern. Med.* **254** (2003) 597-604.

[70] J. Robitaille, D. Gaudet, L. Pérusse *et al.* Features of the metabolic syndrome are modulated by an interaction between the peroxisome proliferator-activated receptor-delta -87T>C polymorphism and dietary fat in French-Canadians. *Int. J. Obes. (Lond).* **31** (2007) 411-417.

[71] J. Aberle, I. Hopfer, F.U. Beil *et al.* Association of the T+294C polymorphism in PPAR delta with low HDL cholesterol and coronary heart disease risk in women. *Int. J. Med. Sci.* **3** (2006) 108-111.

[72]   J. Aberle, I. Hopfer, F.U. Beil *et al.* Association of peroxisome proliferator-activated receptor delta +294T/C with body mass index and interaction with peroxisome proliferator-activated receptor alpha L162V. *Int. J. Obes. (Lond).* **30** (2006) 1709-1713.

[73]   M. Vänttinen, P. Nuutila, T. Kuulasmaa *et al.* Single nucleotide polymorphisms in the peroxisome proliferator-activated receptor delta gene are associated with skeletal muscle glucose uptake. *Diabetes* **54** (2005) 3587-3591.

[74]   A.J. Hautala, A.S. Leon, J.S. Skinner *et al.* Peroxisome proliferator-activated receptor-delta polymorphisms are associated with physical performance and plasma lipids: the HERITAGE Family Study. *Am. J. Physiol. Heart Circ. Physiol.* **292** (2007) H2498-H2505.

[75]   L. Andrulionyte, P. Peltola, J.L. Chiasson *et al.* Single nucleotide polymorphisms of PPARD in combination with the Gly482Ser substitution of PGC-1A and the Pro12Ala substitution of PPARG2 predict the conversion from impaired glucose tolerance to type 2 diabetes: the STOP-NIDDM trial. *Diabetes* **55** (2006) 2148-2152.

[76]   B.K. Pedersen and C.P. Fischer. Physiological roles of muscle-derived interleukin-6 in response to exercise. *Curr. Opin. Clin. Nutr. Metab. Care* **10** (2007) 265-271.

[77]   K. Yoshida, T. Shimizugawa, M. Ono *et al.* Angiopoietin-like protein 4 is a potent hyperlipidemia-inducing factor in mice and inhibitor of lipoprotein lipase. *J. Lipid Res.* **43** (2002) 1770-1772.

[78]   H. Ge, G. Yang, X. Yu *et al.* Oligomerization state-dependent hyperlipidemic effect of angiopoietin-like protein 4. *J. Lipid Res.* **45** (2004) 2071-2079.

[79]   A. Xu, M.C. Lam, K.W. Chan *et al.* Angiopoietin-like protein 4 decreases blood glucose and improves glucose tolerance but induces hyperlipidemia and hepatic steatosis in mice. *Proc. Natl. Acad. Sci. U.S.A.* **102** (2005) 6086-6091.

[80]   A. Köster, Y.B. Chao, M. Mosior *et al.* Transgenic angiopoietin-like (angptl)4 overexpression and targeted disruption of angptl4 and angptl3: regulation of triglyceride metabolism. *Endocrinology* **146** (2005) 4943-4950.

[81]   X. Yu, S.C. Burgess, H. Ge *et al.* Inhibition of cardiac lipoprotein utilization by transgenic overexpression of Angptl4 in the heart. *Proc. Natl. Acad. Sci. U.S.A.* **102** (2005) 1767-1772.

[82]   S. Mandard, F. Zandbergen, E. van Straten *et al.* The fasting-induced adipose factor/angiopoietin-like protein 4 is physically associated with lipoproteins and governs plasma lipid levels and adiposity. *J. Biol. Chem.* **281** (2006) 934-944. Erratum in: *J. Biol. Chem.* **281** (2006) 21575.

Nuclear Receptors as Molecular Targets for Cardiometabolic and Central Nervous System Diseases   61
J.L. Junien and B. Staels (Eds.)
IOS Press, 2008

New Insights in the Role of the Intestine in Reverse Cholesterol Transport

Folkert Kuipers
Laboratory of Pediatrics, Center for Liver, Digestive, and Metabolic Diseases, University Medical Center Groningen, Hanzeplein 1, 9700 RB Groningen, The Netherlands

Abstract. The liver is considered the major "control center" for maintenance of whole-body cholesterol homeostasis. This organ is the main site for *de novo* cholesterol synthesis, clearing cholesterol-containing chylomicron remnants and low-density lipoprotein (LDL) particles from plasma and is the major contributor to high-density lipoprotein (HDL) formation. The liver has a central position in the classical definition of the reverse cholesterol transport pathway by taking up periphery-derived cholesterol from lipoprotein particles followed by conversion into bile acids or its direct secretion into bile for eventual removal via the feces. During the past couple of years, however, an additional important role of the intestine in maintenance of cholesterol homeostasis and regulation of plasma cholesterol levels has become apparent. Firstly, molecular mechanisms of cholesterol absorption have been elucidated and novel pharmacological compounds have been identified that interfere with the process and positively impact plasma cholesterol levels. Secondly, it is now evident that the intestine itself contributes to fecal neutral sterol loss as a cholesterol-secreting organ: selective modulation of this process may provide an effective means to accelerate cholesterol turnover. Finally, very recent work has unequivocally demonstrated that the intestine contributes significantly to plasma HDL cholesterol levels and that intestine-specific activation of LXR leads to "clinically relevant" elevation of plasma HDL levels in animal models. Thus, the intestine is a potential target for novel anti-atherosclerotic treatment strategies that, in addition to interference with cholesterol absorption, modulate direct cholesterol excretion and plasma HDL cholesterol levels.

Keywords. Enterocyte-ABC transporters, Liver X Receptor, bile salts, high-density lipoproteins

Introduction

Maintenance of cholesterol homeostasis in the body requires accurate metabolic cross-talk between processes that govern *de novo* cholesterol synthesis and turnover to adequately cope with (large) fluctuations in dietary cholesterol intake. Imbalance may lead to elevated plasma cholesterol levels and increased risk for cardiovascular diseases (CVD), the main cause of death in Western society. A multitude of epidemiological studies has shown the direct link between high plasma cholesterol, particularly of low-density lipoprotein (LDL) cholesterol, and risk for CVD. Treatment of high plasma cholesterol has been focused for many years on interference with cholesterol synthesis by application of statins. Statins are competitive inhibitors of 3-hydroxy-3-methylglutaryl coenzyme A (HMG-CoA) reductase, the rate-controlling enzyme in the cholesterol biosynthesis pathway. Inhibition of cholesterol synthesis leads to reduced production of very-low-density lipoprotein (VLDL) particles by the liver and particularly, up-regulation of LDL receptor activity. Both processes contribute to lowering of plasma LDL cholesterol levels [1]. Large clinical trials have established the beneficial effects of statin treatment [2]. However, a relative large number of hypercholesterolemic patients do not adequately respond to statin therapy or remain at risk for CVD despite substantial reductions in LDL cholesterol. Consequently, alternative strategies are currently actively pursued, particularly high-density lipoprotein (HDL)-raising approaches. These approaches are considered particularly promising, as data from epidemiological studies indicate that every 1 mg/dL increase in HDL cholesterol reduces CVD risk by 2%-3% [3]. In addition, strategies aiming at interference with intestinal cholesterol metabolism are gaining interest. A major development has been the introduction of ezetimibe, a potent inhibitor of intestinal cholesterol absorption that reduces plasma LDL cholesterol by approximately 20% in mildly hypercholesterolemic patients [4]. Likewise, phytosterol/stanol (esters)-enriched functional foods have successfully been introduced for lowering of plasma cholesterol levels through interference with cholesterol absorption [5].

Recently obtained insights in intestinal cholesterol trafficking may open even more promising avenues for further developments. It appears that the intestine actively excretes cholesterol and thereby, significantly contributes to fecal sterol excretion. In addition, it appears that the intestine is an important source of HDL cholesterol, also known as "good" cholesterol. Thus, the intestine is an attractive target for new therapeutic strategies aimed to alter plasma cholesterol profiles and to reduce the risk for CVD. This review summarizes the important new findings regarding the mechanism(s) of intestinal cholesterol absorption, with specific focus on newly identified transporter proteins, the novel concept of direct intestinal cholesterol secretion and the role of the intestine in HDL biogenesis.

Some Basic Features of Cholesterol

Cholesterol is essential for mammalian life as a structural component of cellular membranes, influencing membrane organization and thereby membrane properties [6]. Cholesterol is the precursor molecule of steroid hormones and therefore, essential for metabolic control. Accumulation of free cholesterol, rather than cholesteryl esters, has been shown to induce apoptosis in macrophages [7]. Thus, cholesterol is a key component in cellular and whole-body physiology and cholesterol homeostasis is tightly regulated at a variety of levels.

Body cholesterol derives from two sources, i.e. *de novo* biosynthesis and diet. The rate-controlling enzyme in the synthetic pathway is HMG-CoA reductase, a highly regulated enzyme that catalyses the conversion of HMG-CoA into mevalonate. Cholesterol itself regulates feedback inhibition of HMG-CoA reductase activity, as accumulation of sterols in the endoplasmic reticulum (ER) membrane triggers HMG-CoA reductase to bind to Insig proteins, which leads to ubiquitination and degradation of HMG-CoA reductase [8]. In addition, cholesterol regulates the gene expression of HMG-CoA reductase indirectly by blocking the activation of the transcription factor sterol regulatory element-binding protein-2 (SREBP-2) [9].

The contribution of the two sources to the total pool of cholesterol differs between species and prevailing diet composition, but the total cholesterol pool is similar in rodents and humans when expressed on the basis of body weight [10]. Cholesterol synthesis in the liver is highly sensitive to the amount of (dietary) cholesterol that reaches the liver from the intestine via the chylomicron-remnant pathway. The Western-type human diet provides approximately 400 mg of cholesterol per day. On top of this, the liver secretes approximately 1 gram of cholesterol into bile per day. Intestinal cholesterol absorption efficiency in humans is highly variable, ranging from 15% to 85% in healthy subjects [11]. After uptake by enterocytes, cholesterol is packed with triglycerides into chylomicrons and secreted into the lymph. In the circulation, the triglycerides are rapidly hydrolyzed and free fatty acids are taken up by the peripheral tissues. Cholesterol-enriched chylomicron remnants are subsequently cleared by the liver. Since chylomicron remnants, which contain most of the cholesterol that is being absorbed from the intestine, are rapidly taken up by the liver, interference with the absorption process directly influences hepatic cholesterol metabolism.

The healthy liver is perfectly equipped for handling large amounts of cholesterol. When relatively large amounts of cholesterol reach the liver, *de novo* synthesis and LDL uptake are rapidly down-regulated. In addition, the liver can dispose excess cholesterol molecules in several ways. A rapid response involves esterification of cholesterol by acyl CoA cholesterol acyltransferase (ACAT) 2 for storage as cholesterylesters in cytoplasmic lipid droplets. Cholesterylester can be hydrolyzed when necessary and this esterification/hydrolysis cycle provides cells with short-term buffering capacity for cholesterol. The liver, like the intestine, is able to produce and secrete VLDL particles, which consist of a neutral lipid core composed of cholesterylesters and triacylglycerols and a monolayer surface containing phospholipids, free cholesterol, and a variety of apolipoproteins. Finally, cholesterol can be converted into bile acids by the hepatocytes, followed by their secretion into the bile along with significant amounts of free cholesterol and phosphatidylcholine. In humans, cholesterol lost via the feces consists of approximately 50% acidic (= bile acids) and 50% neutral sterols, emphasizing the point that conversion into bile acids represents a major pathway for cholesterol elimination.

Peripheral cells, e.g. macrophages, muscle and fat cells, are not able to form lipoproteins or to metabolize cholesterol extensively. Therefore, these cell-types depend massively on efflux pathways for removal of their excess cholesterol. It is generally assumed that HDL is the primary acceptor for cholesterol efflux from cells. HDL cholesterol can subsequently be taken up by the liver for further processing. This pathway is generally referred to as the Reverse Cholesterol Transport (RCT) pathway. The RCT pathway is particularly important for removal of excess cholesterol from macrophages, as accumulation of esterified cholesterol in these cells is considered a primary step in the development of atherosclerosis. Several epidemiological studies have shown that plasma HDL is an independent, negative risk factor for the development of CVD. The common hypothesis is that high HDL cholesterol levels decrease the risk for CVD by removing the excess of cholesterol from the macrophages and enhancing RCT. Recent work, however, indicates that this is an oversimplification and that current concepts of RCT require re-definition [12]. In addition, the anti-inflammatory and anti-oxidant features of molecules rather than cholesterol associated with the HDL particles, like paraoxonase, platelet activating factor-acetylhydrolase or lysophospholipids, are becoming increasingly apparent.

Towards Understanding of Intestinal Cholesterol Absorption

In the past years, insight in regulation of cholesterol absorption has greatly increased by identification of transporter proteins involved. In addition, unraveling of molecular regulation of their expression is progressing. Yet, it should be realized that besides transporter proteins, the presence of bile acids in the intestinal lumen is an essential prerequisite for absorption to occur [13].

Identification of Novel Proteins Involved in Cholesterol Absorption

Cholesterol absorption has long been considered a merely passive process, despite the fact that the process is clearly selective since dietary cholesterol is absorbed with a relative high efficiency whereas structurally similar phytosterols are not. Several candidate intestinal cholesterol transporters have been proposed during the past couple of years, e.g. SR-BI [14] and aminopeptidase N [15], but their role (if any) has remained elusive so far. The recent identification of the Niemann-Pick C1 like 1 (NPC1L1) protein as a crucial molecule involved in cholesterol uptake by enterocytes [16] and of Abcg5 and Abcg8 proteins as (intestinal) cholesterol efflux transporters [17-19], has provided definite proof that cholesterol absorption is a protein-mediated, selective and active process.

The identification of NPC1L1 is strongly facilitated by the discovery of a powerful cholesterol absorption inhibitor, i.e. ezetimibe [20]. Ezetimibe and analogs comprise a new class of sterol absorption inhibitors that reduce diet-induced hypercholesterolemia in mice, hamsters, rats, rabbits, dogs, monkeys and humans. Using a bioinformatics approach, Altmann *et al* [16] have identified the NPC1L1 protein as a putative cholesterol transporter in intestinal cells. NPC1L1 is expressed in the intestine at the brush border membrane and *Npc1l*-deficient mice show a 69% reduction in fractional cholesterol absorption. Importantly, treatment with ezetimibe could not further reduce fractional cholesterol absorption efficiency in these mice, indicating that NPC1L1 at least is involved in a pathway targeted by ezetimibe. In support of this, recent studies have shown that ezetimibe glucuronide, the active molecule, indeed binds to cells expressing NPC1L1 [21]. The exact cellular localization of NPC1L1 is, however, still under debate. Iyer *et al* [22] showed that NPC1L1 is glycosylated and enriched in the BBM of rat enterocytes. Davies *et al* [23] who were the first to identify NPC1L1 as a homolog of the Niemann-Pick type C (NPC) protein, showed in HepG2 cells that NPC1L1 is localized to a subcellular vesicular compartment but not in the plasma membrane. Using immortalized fibroblasts from wild-type and *Npc1l1* knock-out mice these authors also showed that lack of NPC1L1 activity causes dysregulation of caveolin transport and localization, suggesting that the observed sterol transport defect may be an indirect result of the inability of *Npc1l1*-deficient cells to properly target and/or regulate cholesterol transport in the cells.

Another possible mechanism of action of ezetimibe has been proposed by Smart and colleagues [24]. These authors described the presence of a stable complex of annexin (ANX) 2 and caveolin (CAV) 1 located in enterocytes of zebrafish and mouse. Disruption of this complex by morpholino antisense oligonucleotides in zebrafish could prevent normal uptake of cholesterol. Ezetimibe treatment of zebrafish, C57BL/6 mice fed a Western-type diet and LDL receptor knock-out mice disrupts the ANX2-CAV1 complex, suggesting that ANX2 and CAV1 are components of an intestinal sterol transport complex and targets for ezetimibe. Recent research using CAV1-deficient mice revealed, however, that inhibition of cholesterol absorption by ezetimibe does not require the presence of CAV1 [25]. In addition, rabbits do not appear to form the ANX2-CAV1 complexes, yet, their cholesterol absorption efficiency is still inhibited by ezetimibe [26].

Other proteins critical in control of sterol absorption are the ATP-binding cassette (ABC) transporter proteins, G5 and G8. ABCG5 and ABCG8 act as functional heterodimers [27] and are localized at the canalicular membrane of hepatocytes and at the brush border membrane of enterocytes. Mutations in the human genes encoding ABCG5 or ABCG8 have been shown to cause the inherited disease sitosterolemia [17-19], which is characterized by an accumulation of plant sterols (e.g. sitosterol, campesterol) in blood and tissues due to their enhanced intestinal absorption and decreased biliary removal. Thus, ABCG5/ABCG8 limit plant sterol absorption by effective efflux back into the intestinal lumen. Since ABCG5/ABCG8 also accommodate cholesterol, as evidenced from the fact that *Abcg5/g8*-deficient mice show a strongly reduced biliary cholesterol secretion [28]. This system also provides a means to control cholesterol absorption efficiency. Yet, *Abcg5* and/or *Abcg8* deficiency in mice clearly enhances phytosterol absorption [29-31], but reported effects on cholesterol absorption efficiency are minimal [28,29]. On the other hand, over-expression of *ABCG5* and *ABCG8* in mice as well as pharmacological induction of their expression lead to a strongly decreased fractional cholesterol absorption [31,32], indicating that ABCG5 and ABCG8 play a role in control of cholesterol absorption under certain conditions.

Other transporter proteins, like the scavenger receptor BI (SR-BI) and ABCA1 have been suggested to play a role in control of cholesterol absorption. In the small intestine, SR-BI is localized both at the apical membrane and at the basolateral membrane of enterocytes, with different expression levels along the length of the small intestine [13]. It was reported that mice deficient in SR-BI show only a small increase in fractional cholesterol absorption efficiency and a small decrease in fecal neutral sterol output [33]. On the other hand, intestine-specific over-expression of SR-BI in mice leads to increased cholesterol absorption in short-term experiments [34], indicating that SR-BI might have a role in the process.

Although earlier reports [35] have suggested an apical localization, it is evident that ABCA1 is localized at the basolateral membranes of enterocytes [36,37]. The conflicting results yielded in studies assessing intestinal cholesterol absorption in mice lacking Abca1 [38,39], suggest that the overall effect of Abca1 on absorption is very minor. However, as will be described later, this protein does have an important function in intestinal cholesterol metabolism.

After uptake, cholesterol is esterified by the enzyme ACAT2 in the endoplasmic reticulum (ER) of enterocytes. It was reported that *Acat2*-deficiency in mice on a low-cholesterol chow diet does not affect cholesterol absorption efficiency, however, *Acat2*-deficient mice show a clear reduction in cholesterol absorption upon feeding a high-fat/high-cholesterol diet and as a consequence, are resistant to diet-induced hypercholesterolemia [40]. Other proteins crucial for cholesterol absorption are those involved in chylomicron formation, like apolipoprotein B (ApoB) and microsomal triglyceride transfer protein (MTP), and proteins involved in intracellular chylomicron trafficking such as SARA2. These proteins will not be further discussed.

The major routes of cholesterol in enterocytes and the proteins involved are depicted schematically in Figure 1.

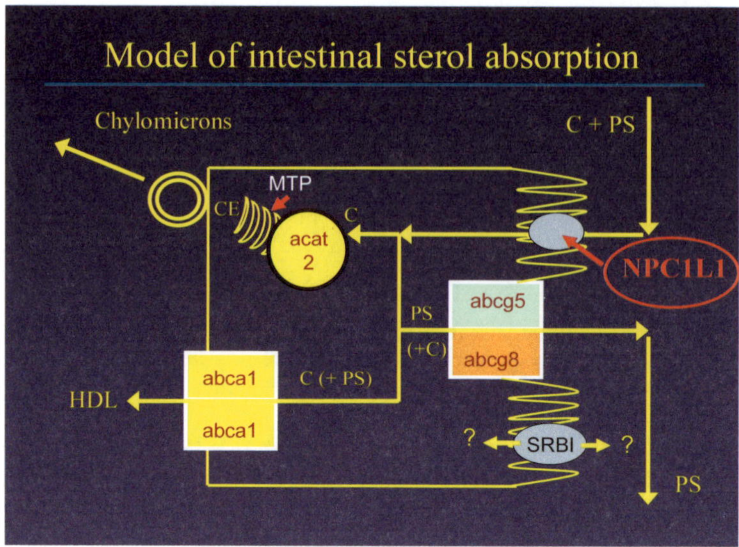

Figure 1. Schematic overview of the major routes of cholesterol in enterocytes. Dietary and biliary cholesterol are taken up via the action of NPC1L1. In the ER, cholesterol is esterified and incorporated into chylomicrons, which are subsequently secreted into lymph. Non-esterified sterols can be re-secreted into the intestinal lumen via the action of ABCG5/G8 or secreted towards ApoA1 via the action of ABCA1.
ABCA1, ABCG5, ABCG8: ATP-binding cassette transporter A1, G5, G8; ACAT2: acyl-coenzyme A:cholesterol acyltransferase 2; C: cholesterol; CE: cholesterylester; ER: endoplasmic reticulum; MTP: microsomal triglyceride transfer protein; NPC1L1: Niemann-Pick C1 like 1 protein.

Regulation of Cholesterol Absorption

As indicated above, cholesterol can be taken up from the intestinal lumen by NPC1L1 and effluxed back into the lumen via ABCG5 and ABCG8. When both processes are active and present in the same cells, a classical futile cycle arises, enabling very sensitive regulation. Interference with this system has a great potential for reducing plasma cholesterol.

Lowering of NPC1L1 expression provides potential means to reduce cholesterol absorption. Mechanisms involved in transcriptional control of NPC1L1 are beginning to be unraveled. The nuclear receptor peroxisome proliferator-activated receptor (PPAR)δ/β (NR1C2) has been shown to decrease cholesterol absorption, presumably by decreasing *NPC1L1* expression [41]. Activation of PPARδ/β by the synthetic agonist GW610742 results in a 43% reduction of cholesterol absorption in mice, which coincides with unchanged intestinal expression of *Abcg5* and *Abcg8* but a decreased intestinal expression of *Npc1l1*. Treatment of human colon-derived Caco-2 cells with ligands for PPARδ/β, but not for PPARγ or PPARα, decreases *NPC1L1* expression as well [41]. Whether PPARδ/β regulates NPC1L1 directly or indirectly via transcriptional repression, is still under investigation.

The major regulatory pathways in cholesterol metabolism are controlled by the nuclear receptor Liver X Receptor (LXR). Two LXR isotypes have been identified in mammals, i.e. LXRα (NR1H3) which is mainly expressed in the liver, kidney, intestine, spleen and adrenals, and LXRβ (NR1H2) which is expressed ubiquitously. Natural ligands for both LXRs are oxysterols. After activation, LXR heterodimerizes with Retinoid X Receptor (RXR) [42]. Activated RXR/LXR heterodimers bind to specific LXR response elements (LXREs) in the promoter regions of their target genes and activate gene transcription. LXR-target genes include many genes involved in cellular cholesterol efflux like *ABCA1*, *ABCG1*, *ABCG5,* and *ABCG8* and genes involved in lipogenesis like sterol regulatory element-binding protein (SREBP)-1C, fatty acid synthase (FAS) and *acetyl-CoA* carboxylase (ACC). Global LXR-activation by synthetic agonists therefore has a plethora of effects including elevated HDL levels, hypertriglyceridemia, hepatic steatosis, increased biliary cholesterol excretion, reduced intestinal cholesterol absorption efficiency and increased neutral sterol loss via the feces [43,44]. The decreased intestinal cholesterol absorption is primarily due to increased cholesterol efflux of cholesterol towards the intestinal lumen due to increased *Abcg5* and *Abcg8* expression, as fractional cholesterol absorption is reduced upon LXR-activation in wild-type mice but remains unaltered in *Abcg5/g8*-deficient mice [29] and *Abcg5*-deficient mice [32] under these conditions. Other mechanisms, such as reduced intestinal *Npc1l1* expression after LXR-activation contribute to reduced cholesterol absorption, as recently shown in *ApoE2* knock-out mice [45].

Dietary phytosterols and phytostanols and their esters have been introduced in functional foods to suppress intestinal cholesterol absorption and hence to reduce the risk for CVD. Phytosterols and stanols are thought to decrease cholesterol absorption by competing with cholesterol for incorporation into mixed micelles in the intestinal lumen. However, several recent studies suggest additional mechanisms involving alterations of intestinal gene expression. Igel and colleagues [46] showed for the first time that phytosterols and stanols are actually taken up by the enterocytes and subsequently re-secreted into the gut lumen, most probably through the action of Abcg5/Abcg8 transporters. This finding indicates that phytosterols and stanols, in addition to modes of action within the intestinal lumen, may exert metabolic actions from inside the enterocytes. Moreover, dietary phytostanol consumption (2.5 g) once a day reduces LDL cholesterol as effective as consumption of 2.5 g phytostanols ingested in three daily portions [47], suggesting that luminal concentrations may not be the key to the control of metabolic actions. The identification of a phytosterol-derived agonist for the nuclear receptor LXR [48] has led to the proposal that phytosterols and stanols decrease cholesterol absorption via activation of intestinal LXR. Recent *in vivo* studies, however, showed that dietary phytosterols and phytostanols decrease cholesterol absorption without activating LXR in rodent models: e.g. Plosch *et al* [49] showed that addition of 0.5% phytostanols/sterols to a semi-synthetic diet did not affect intestinal expression of *ABC transporters* and *Npc1l1* in C57BL mice. Additionally, these authors showed that the plant sterol/stanol-induced reduction of cholesterol absorption in mice is not influenced by *Abcg5*-deficiency [49], indicating that intra-luminal events are most relevant for the inhibitory effect of these dietary compounds.

Novel Role of the Intestine in Reverse Cholesterol Transport

It is clear that the intestine plays a major role in cholesterol homeostasis as a cholesterol absorbing organ. However, recent studies revealed that the intestine also acts as an excretory organ in the Reverse Cholesterol Transport (RCT) pathway [50]. This pathway is classically defined as the HDL-mediated flux of cholesterol from peripheral cells to the liver, followed by its secretion into bile and disposal via the feces. RCT is extremely important in prevention of CVD as it removes excess cholesterol from macrophages present in the arterial vessel wall. The amount of cholesterol secreted into bile is substantial. As only part of it is absorbed by the intestine, it contributes significantly to cholesterol loss via the feces. However, a novel pathway that contributes to fecal cholesterol loss has recently been established.

Non-dietary cholesterol present in the intestinal lumen consists of a fraction secreted by the liver into the bile and a second fraction directly secreted by the intestine. Measuring dietary cholesterol, cholesterol absorption and cholesterol loss via the feces in patients with complete obstruction of common bile duct due to carcinoma of the head of the pancreas unequivocally established the presence of intestinally secreted cholesterol in the feces [51]. By intestinal perfusion studies in humans, Simmonds *et al* [52] have tried to quantify this route. In a triple lumen tube system, perfusion studies can be carried out using micellar solutions with radio-labeled cholesterol. Decrease in specific activity is interpreted as secretion of endogenous cholesterol from the intestine and the contribution of endogenously secreted cholesterol from the intestine is estimated to be about 44% of total fecal output, but direct proof for the existence of this pathway could not be provided.

Since these early experiments, the focus of research has shifted more towards the liver. Biliary cholesterol and bile acid secretions are believed to represent the major pathways for removal of excess cholesterol. However, recent calculations of cholesterol fluxes in different mouse models again emphasize the relevance of intestinal cholesterol secretion. Plösch and colleagues [44] showed that the pathway of intestinal cholesterol secretion can be induced in mice by treatment with the synthetic LXR-agonist T0901317. In C57BL/6 mice, efflux of cholesterol from the intestinal epithelium into the lumen, calculated from the difference between dietary and biliary input minus fecal output, contributes up to 36% of the total fecal cholesterol loss. Pharmacological LXR-activation in these mice triples the intestinal cholesterol secretion, showing that this represents a valid, inducible pathway for removal of cholesterol in mice.

To further characterize this route, Kruit *et al* [50] have studied the effects of LXR-activation by the synthetic agonist GW3965 in wild-type and *Mdr2*-deficient mice. *Mdr2*-Pgp (or Abcb4 according to the new nomenclature) mediates the ATP-dependent translocation of phospholipids at the canalicular membrane of hepatocytes. Consequently, *Mdr2*-deficiency leads to the inability to secrete phospholipids into the bile. Due to the tight coupling of phospholipid and cholesterol secretion, these mice also show a severely impaired biliary cholesterol secretion [53,54]. Despite the impaired biliary cholesterol secretion, chow-fed *Mdr2*$^{-/-}$ mice show a similar fecal neutral sterols loss as wild-type mice, suggesting that the intestine indeed contributes to the fecal neutral sterol loss. LXR-activation increases fecal neutral sterol output to a similar extent in *Mdr2*$^{-/-}$ and wild-type mice, although biliary cholesterol secretion remains impaired in *Mdr2*$^{-/-}$ mice but increases in wild-type mice. These data show that the increased fecal cholesterol loss upon LXR-activation is independent of biliary cholesterol secretion. Although fractional cholesterol absorption decreases to a greater extent in *Mdr2*$^{-/-}$ mice compared to wild-type mice upon LXR-activation, it could be calculated that at least 57% of fecal cholesterol originates from intestinal secretion in *Mdr2*$^{-/-}$ mice.

The most intriguing question, namely the origin of intestine-derived cholesterol has remained unanswered so far. Part of the cholesterol could, in theory, originate from enhanced sloughing of intestinal cells or reflect a consequence of increased intestinal *de novo* cholesterol synthesis. Upon LXR-activation, however, intestinal *HMG-CoA reductase* gene expression remains unchanged [44,50], indicative for unchanged cholesterol synthesis, while fecal sterol loss increases 3 times. Staining for the proliferation marker Ki-67 has revealed no signs of increased intestinal cell proliferation upon LXR-activation, making the possibility of enhanced cell shedding less likely. Using intravenously injected radio-labeled cholesterol as a marker, Kruit and colleagues [50] additionally showed that fecal loss of plasma-derived cholesterol is 1.7-fold higher upon LXR-activation in *Mdr2*$^{-/-}$ mice, suggesting that the intestine plays an important role independently of biliary cholesterol in cholesterol transport from plasma to the feces.

Further research should be done to identify the putative proteins involved in this pathway. The sterol efflux proteins, ABCG5/ABCG8, seem to be good candidates, as increased fecal neutral sterol output upon LXR-activation requires the presence of Abcg5 and Abcg8 and transgenic mice over-expressing human *ABCG5* and *ABCG8* (*hG5G8Tg*) show significantly increased fecal neutral sterol loss. However, deficiency of *Abcg5* and/or *Abcg8* leads to only mild or no decrease in fecal neutral sterol loss and the increased fecal neutral sterol excretion loss in the *hG5G8Tg* mice is inhibited in *hG5G8Tg* mice lacking *Mdr2* (*Mdr2$^{-/-}$ hG5G8Tg* mice), suggesting that biliary cholesterol secretion is responsible for the increased fecal sterol loss in *hG5G8Tg* mice [55]. However, *hG5G8Tg* mice show a high expression of human *ABCG5* and *ABCG8* in the liver but their expression in the intestine is far less pronounced [31]. Thus, the question whether intestinal ABCG5 and ABCG8 are important for intestinal cholesterol efflux under normal conditions still remains unanswered.

Virtually nothing is known about transporter systems involved in uptake of plasma cholesterol by enterocytes prior to its excretion into the intestinal lumen. LXR-activation can up-regulate a number of cholesterol transporters, of which only SR-BI is known to be involved in cholesterol uptake, at least in the liver. Chow-fed *SR-BI$^{-/-}$* mice show only a small decrease in fecal neutral sterol loss, suggesting a relatively small contribution of intestinal SR-BI to the control of fecal cholesterol excretion. However, basolaterally localized SR-BI in enterocytes could theoretically play a role in cholesterol. When free cholesterol in enterocytes decreases due to activation of ABCG5 and ABCG8, uptake of the sterol from the plasma compartment may become energetically favorable.

Intestinal Contribution to HDL Biogenesis

The intestine along with the liver, has been known for many years to synthesize and secrete apolipoprotein A-I (ApoA-I), the principal apolipoprotein of HDL. Glickman and Green [56] have described the synthesis of ApoA-I by the intestine of rats. Wu and Windmueller [57] reported that intestinally synthesized ApoA-I contributes up to 56% of total plasma ApoA-I in rats and demonstrated that intestine plays a potential role in HDL particle assembly.

In addition to ApoA-I, ATP-binding cassette (ABC) transporter 1 (ABCA1) is of crucial importance for HDL formation. Three different groups have independently reported mutations of the ABCA1 gene as the cause of Tangier disease [58-60]. Tangier disease is characterized by almost complete absence of plasma HDL, abnormal accumulation of cholesteryl esters in reticuloendothelial cells of many tissues and early incidence of atherosclerosis. No abnormalities in the ApoA-I protein or in protein synthesis have been found. These findings and the subsequent generation of *Abca1$^{-/-}$* mice which also lack plasma HDL [39], underscore ABCA1 which is crucial for HDL formation.

ABCA1 performs the rate-controlling step in HDL formation by mediating the efflux of cholesterol and phospholipids to nascent ApoA-I. ABCA1 is widely expressed throughout the body [61], however not all tissues are important for the regulation of plasma HDL. Bone marrow transplantation studies revealed that macrophage expression of *Abca1* contributes only minimally to plasma HDL [62]. Macrophage ABCA1 is, however, important for the development of atherosclerosis because deficiency of *Abca1* in bone marrow-derived cells increases the susceptibility to atherosclerosis in sensitive strains of mice [63]. Conversely, over-expression of *ABCA1* in bone marrow-derived cells inhibits the progression of atherosclerotic lesions in such mice [64].

As both the liver and intestine synthesize ApoA-I and express significant levels of ABCA1, they are prone to contribute to biogenesis of plasma HDL levels. Studies employing adenoviral *Abca1* transfer to mouse liver *in vivo* [65,66] showed that treatment of C57BL/6 mice with adenovirus containing *rABCA1-GFP* results in a 2-fold increase in plasma HDL levels. Wellington *et al* [66] treated mice with increasing doses of *ABCA1*-containing adenoviruses, which results in a dose-dependent increase in hepatic ABCA1 protein expression. Liver-specific *Abca1* knock-down by 50% in mice using siRNA results in a 40% decrease of plasma HDL cholesterol levels, indicating that hepatic *Abca1* expression correlates with plasma HDL levels in mice [67].

The liver is the major contributor to plasma HDL as liver-specific deficiency of *Abca1* results in a decrease of plasma HDL cholesterol levels by ~80%. *In vivo* catabolism of HDL ApoA-I isolated from wild-type mice is 2-fold higher in $Abca1^{-L/-L}$ mice due to a 2-fold higher rate of catabolism of ApoA-I in the kidneys [68]. These data unequivocally demonstrate that hepatic *Abca1* is responsible for the maintenance of the circulating plasma HDL by direct lipidation of lipid-poor ApoA-1 containing particles. These data also show that, although the liver is the major organ responsible for HDL levels, additional extra-hepatic sites also contribute to HDL biogenesis.

To address the contribution of intestinal *Abca1* to plasma HDL, intestine-specific *Abca1* knock-out ($Abca1^{-i/-i}$) mice have been created using the Cre/Lox system with the Cre transgene under the control of the villin promoter [69]. Intestinal *Abca1* deficiency results in a 30% decrease in plasma HDL cholesterol levels, indicating that intestinal *Abca1* is critically involved in HDL biogenesis. Combined deletion of both hepatic and intestinal *Abca1* results in a 90% decrease of plasma HDL, which is similar to the level found in the whole-body $Abca1^{-/-}$ mice, proving that the liver and intestine are really the two major sites for HDL biogenesis. Absence of intestinal *Abca1* results in decreased transport of dietary cholesterol into plasma HDL, but total intestinal cholesterol absorption is not affected. Surprisingly, lymphatic HDL content is hardly affected in $Abca1^{-i/-i}$ mice. In contrast, HDL is virtually absent in lymph of $Abca1^{-L/-L}$ mice, indicating that lymph HDL originates from the plasma compartment rather than directly from the intestine [69]. This finding has solved a long-lasting debate on the origin of lymphatic HDL. It would be interesting to see whether lack of intestinal *Abca1* influences the development of atherosclerosis.

Modulation of Plasma HDL by Intestine-specific LXR-activation

As discussed above, LXR is a major regulator of cholesterol metabolism and LXR-agonists are considered promising candidates for novel treatment strategies against atherosclerosis. Indeed, treatment of $ApoE^{-/-}$ and $LDLr^{-/-}$ mice, both are sensitive to atherosclerosis development, with synthetic LXR-agonists inhibits development of atherosclerosis [70,71]. However, general LXR-activation also leads to increased lipogenesis, hypertriglyceridemia and hepatic steatosis in rodents and is therefore not recommended for use in humans. Specific LXR-activation in the intestine may be beneficial in this respect, as it can theoretically lead to decreased cholesterol absorption, increased intestinal cholesterol excretion and plasma HDL levels. Recent data from our laboratory, using a relative intestine-specific LXR-agonist in the various *Abca1* knock-out models described above, indeed showed that induction of intestinal *Abca1* expression only has the desired effect without adverse effects on triglyceride metabolism [72].

Conclusion

During the past 5 years, a number of developments have greatly contributed to appreciation of the important role of the intestine in maintenance of cholesterol homeostasis, including identification of transporter proteins involved in uptake and secretion of cholesterol by enterocytes, establishment of the direct cholesterol excretion pathway of the intestine, definition of the role of the intestine in HDL biogenesis.

A wealth of data indicate that the intestine should be considered a promising target for development of anti-atherosclerotic drugs that, in addition to interference with cholesterol absorption, may directly modulate cholesterol excretion and plasma HDL cholesterol levels.

References

[1] M.S. Brown and J.L. Goldstein. A receptor-mediated pathway for cholesterol homeostasis. *Science* **232** (1986) 34-47.

[2] H.T. Ong. The statin studies: from targeting hypercholesterolaemia to targeting the high-risk patient. *QJM* **98** (2005) 599-614.

[3] T. Gordon, W.B. Kannel, W.P. Castelli *et al.* Lipoproteins, cardiovascular disease, and death. The Framingham study. *Arch. Intern. Med.* **141** (1981) 1128-1131.

[4] T. Sudhop, D. Lutjohann, A. Kodal *et al.* Inhibition of intestinal cholesterol absorption by ezetimibe in humans. *Circulation* **106** (2002) 1943-1948.

[5] T.A. Miettinen, P. Puska, H. Gylling *et al.* E. Reduction of serum cholesterol with sitostanol-ester margarine in a mildly hypercholesterolemic population. *N. Engl. J. Med.* **333** (1995) 1308-1312. Comment in: *N. Engl. J. Med.* **333** (1995) 1350-1351.

[6] F.R. Maxfield and I. Tabas. Role of cholesterol and lipid organization in disease. *Nature* **438** (2005) 612-621

[7] P.M. Yao and I. Tabas. Free cholesterol loading of macrophages induces apoptosis involving the fas pathway. *J. Biol. Chem.* **275** (2000) 23807-23813.

[8] N. Sever, T. Yang, M.S. Brown *et al.* Accelerated degradation of HMG CoA reductase mediated by binding of insig-1 to its sterol-sensing domain. *Mol. Cell* **11** (2003) 25-33.

[9] J.L. Goldstein, R.A. DeBose-Boyd, M.S. Brown. Protein sensors for membrane sterols. *Cell* **124** (2006) 35-46.

[10] J.M. Dietschy and S.D. Turley. Control of cholesterol turnover in the mouse. *J. Biol. Chem.* **277** (2002) 3801-3804.

[11] S.M. Grundy. Absorption and metabolism of dietary cholesterol. *Annu. Rev. Nutr.* **3** (1983) 71-96.

[12] A.K. Groen, R.P. Oude Elferink, H.J. Verkade *et al.* The ins and outs of reverse cholesterol transport. *Ann. Med.* **36** (2004) 135-145.

[13] P.J. Voshol, M. Schwarz, A. Rigotti *et al.* Down-regulation of intestinal scavenger receptor class B, type 1 (SR-B1) expression in rodents under conditions of deficient bile delivery to the intestine. *Biochem. J.* **356** (2001) 317-325.

[14] H. Hauser, J.H. Dyer, A. Nandy *et al.* Identification of a receptor mediating absorption of dietary cholesterol in the intestine. *Biochemistry* **37** (1998) 17843-17850.

[15] W. Kramer, F. Girbig, D. Corsiero *et al.* Aminopeptidase N (CD13) is a molecular target of the cholesterol absorption inhibitor ezetimibe in the enterocyte brush border membrane. *J. Biol. Chem.* **280** (2005) 1306-1320.

[16] S.W. Altmann, H.R. Davis, L.J. Zhu *et al.* Niemann-Pick C1 Like 1 protein is critical for intestinal cholesterol absorption. *Science* **303** (2004) 1201-1204.

[17] K. Lu, M.H. Lee, S. Hazard *et al.* Two genes that map to the STSL locus cause sitosterolemia: genomic structure and spectrum of mutations involving sterolin-1 and sterolin-2, encoded by ABCG5 and ABCG8, respectively. *Am. J. Hum. Genet.* **69** (2001) 278-290.

[18] M.H. Lee, K. Lu, S. Hazard *et al.* Identification of a gene, ABCG5, important in the regulation of dietary cholesterol absorption. *Nat. Genet.* **27** (2001) 79-83.

[19] K.E. Berge, H. Tian, G.A. Graf *et al.* Accumulation of dietary cholesterol in sitosterolemia caused by mutations in adjacent ABC transporters. *Science* **290** (2000) 1771-1775. Comment in: *Science* **290** (2000) 1709-1711.

[20] B.G. Salisbury, H.R. Davis, R.E. Burrier *et al.* Hypocholesterolemic activity of a novel inhibitor of cholesterol absorption, SCH 48461. *Atherosclerosis* **115** (1995) 45-63.

[21] M. Garcia-Calvo, J. Lisnock, H.G. Bull *et al.* The target of ezetimibe is Niemann-Pick C1-Like 1 (NPC1L1). *Proc. Natl. Acad. Sci. U.S.A.* **102** (2005) 8132-8137.

[22] S.P. Iyer, X. Yao, J.H. Crona *et al.* Characterization of the putative native and recombinant rat sterol transporter Niemann-Pick C1 Like 1 (NPC1L1) protein. *Biochim. Biophys. Acta* **1722** (2005) 282-292.

[23]   J.P. Davies, B. Levy, Y.A. Ioannou. Evidence for a Niemann-pick C (NPC) gene family: identification and characterization of NPC1L1. *Genomics* **65** (2000) 137-145.

[24]   E.J. Smart, R.A. De Rose, S.A. Farber. Annexin 2-caveolin 1 complex is a target of ezetimibe and regulates intestinal cholesterol transport. *Proc. Natl. Acad. Sci. U.S.A.* **101** (2004) 3450-3455.

[25]   M.A. Valasek, J. Weng, P.W. Shaul *et al.* Caveolin-1 is not required for murine intestinal cholesterol transport. *J. Biol. Chem.* **280** (2005) 28103-28109.

[26]   W. Kramer, D. Corsiero, F. Girbig *et al.* Rabbit small intestine does not contain an annexin II/caveolin 1 complex as a target for 2-azetidinone cholesterol absorption inhibitors. *Biochim. Biophys. Acta* **1758** (2006) 45-54.

[27]   G.A. Graf, W.P. Li, R.D. Gerard *et al.* Coexpression of ATP-binding cassette proteins ABCG5 and ABCG8 permits their transport to the apical surface. *J. Clin. Invest.* **110** (2002) 659-669. Comment in: *J. Clin. Invest.* **110** (2002) 605-609.

[28]   L. Yu, R.E. Hammer, J. Li-Hawkins *et al.* Disruption of Abcg5 and Abcg8 in mice reveals their crucial role in biliary cholesterol secretion. *Proc. Natl. Acad. Sci. U.S.A.* **99** (2002) 16237-16242.

[29]   T. Plösch, V.W. Bloks, Y. Terasawa *et al.* Sitosterolemia in ABC-transporter G5-deficient mice is aggravated on activation of the liver-X receptor. *Gastroenterology* **126** (2004) 290-300.

[30]   E.L. Klett, K. Lu, A. Kosters *et al.* A mouse model of sitosterolemia: absence of Abcg8/sterolin-2 results in failure to secrete biliary cholesterol. *BMC Med.* **2** (2004) 5.

[31]   L. Yu, J. Li-Hawkins, R.E. Hammer *et al.* Overexpression of ABCG5 and ABCG8 promotes biliary cholesterol secretion and reduces fractional absorption of dietary cholesterol. *J. Clin. Invest.* **110** (2002) 671-680. Comment in: *J. Clin. Invest.* **110** (2002) 605-609; *Hepatology* **37** (2003) 940-942.

[32]   L. Yu, J. York, K. von Bergmann *et al.* Stimulation of cholesterol excretion by the liver X receptor agonist requires ATP-binding cassette transporters G5 and G8. *J. Biol. Chem.* **278** (2003) 15565-15570.

[33]   P. Mardones, V. Quiñones, L. Amigo *et al.* Hepatic cholesterol and bile acid metabolism and intestinal cholesterol absorption in scavenger receptor class B type I-deficient mice. *J. Lipid Res.* **42** (2001) 170-180.

[34]   F. Bietrix, D. Yan, M. Nauze *et al.* Accelerated lipid absorption in mice overexpressing intestinal SR-BI. *J. Biol. Chem.* **281** (2006) 7214-7219.

[35]   J.J. Repa, S.D. Turley, J.A. Lobaccaro *et al.* Regulation of absorption and ABC1-mediated efflux of cholesterol by RXR heterodimers. *Science* **289** (2000) 1524-1529. Comment in: *Science* **289** (2000) 1446-1447.

[36]   J.D. Mulligan, M.T. Flowers, A. Tebon *et al.* ABCA1 is essential for efficient basolateral cholesterol efflux during the absorption of dietary cholesterol in chickens. *J. Biol. Chem.* **278** (2003) 13356-13366.

[37]   T. Ohama, K. Hirano, Z. Zhang *et al.* Dominant expression of ATP-binding cassette transporter-1 on basolateral surface of Caco-2 cells stimulated by LXR/RXR ligands. *Biochem. Biophys. Res. Commun.* **296** (2002) 625-630.

[38]   W. Drobnik, B. Lindenthal, B. Lieser *et al.* ATP-binding cassette transporter A1 (ABCA1) affects total body sterol metabolism. *Gastroenterology* **120** (2001) 1203-1211.

[39]   J. McNeish, R.J. Aiello, D. Guyot *et al.* High density lipoprotein deficiency and foam cell accumulation in mice with targeted disruption of ATP-binding cassette transporter-1. *Proc. Natl. Acad. Sci. U.S.A.* **97** (2000) 4245-4250.

[40]   K.K. Buhman, M. Accad, S. Novak *et al.* Resistance to diet-induced hypercholesterolemia and gallstone formation in ACAT2-deficient mice. *Nat. Med.* **6** (2000) 1341-1347.

[41]   J.N. van der Veen, J.K. Kruit, R. Havinga *et al.* Reduced cholesterol absorption upon PPARdelta activation coincides with decreased intestinal expression of NPC1L1. *J. Lipid Res.* **46** (2005) 526-534.

[42]   B.A. Janowski, P.J. Willy, T.R. Devi *et al.* An oxysterol signalling pathway mediated by the nuclear receptor LXR alpha. *Nature* **383** (1996) 728-731.

[43]   A. Grefhorst, B.M. Elzinga, P.J. Voshol *et al.* Stimulation of lipogenesis by pharmacological activation of the liver X receptor leads to production of large, triglyceride-rich very low density lipoprotein particles. *J. Biol. Chem.* **277** (2002) 34182-34190.

[44]   T. Plösch, T. Kok, V.W. Bloks *et al.* Increased hepatobiliary and fecal cholesterol excretion upon activation of the liver X receptor is independent of ABCA1. *J. Biol. Chem.* **277** (2002) 33870-33877.

[45]   C. Duval, V. Touche, A. Tailleux *et al.* Niemann-Pick C1 like 1 gene expression is down-regulated by LXR activators in the intestine. *Biochem. Biophys. Res. Commun.* **340** (2006) 1259-1263.

[46]   M. Igel, U. Giesa, D. Lutjohann *et al.* Comparison of the intestinal uptake of cholesterol, plant sterols, and stanols in mice. *J. Lipid Res.* **44** (2003) 533-538.

[47]   J. Plat, E.N. van Onselen, M.M. van Heugten *et al.* Effects on serum lipids, lipoproteins and fat soluble antioxidant concentrations of consumption frequency of margarines and shortenings enriched with plant stanol esters. *Eur. J. Clin. Nutr.* **54** (2000) 671-677.

[48]   E. Kaneko, M. Matsuda, Y. Yamada *et al.* Induction of intestinal ATP-binding cassette transporters by a phytosterol-derived liver X receptor agonist. *J. Biol. Chem.* **278** (2003) 36091-36098.

[49]   T. Plösch, J.K. Kruit, V.W. Bloks *et al.* Reduction of cholesterol absorption by dietary plant sterols and stanols in mice is independent of the Abcg5/8 transporter. *J. Nutr.* **136** (2006) 2135-2140.

[50]   J.K. Kruit, T. Plösch, R. Havinga *et al.* Increased fecal neutral sterol loss upon liver X receptor activation is independent of biliary sterol secretion in mice. *Gastroenterology* **128** (2005) 147-156.

[51]   S.H. Cheng and M.M. Stanley. Secretion of cholesterol by intestinal mucosa in patients with complete common bile duct obstruction. *Proc. Soc. Exp. Biol. Med.* **101** (1959) 223-225.

[52]   W.J. Simmonds, A.F. Hofmann, E. Theodor. Absorption of cholesterol from a micellar solution: intestinal perfusion studies in man. *J. Clin. Invest.* **46** (1967) 874-890.

[53]   R.P. Oude Elferink, R. Ottenhoff, M. van Wijland *et al.* Uncoupling of biliary phospholipid and cholesterol secretion in mice with reduced expression of mdr2 P-glycoprotein. *J. Lipid Res.* **37** (1996) 1065-1075.

[54]   J.J. Smit, A.H. Schinkel, R.P. Oude Elferink *et al.* Homozygous disruption of the murine mdr2 P-glycoprotein gene leads to a complete absence of phospholipid from bile and to liver disease. *Cell* **75** (1993) 451-462.

[55]   S. Langheim, L. Yu, K. von Bergmann *et al.* ABCG5 and ABCG8 require MDR2 for secretion of cholesterol into bile. *J. Lipid Res.* **46** (2005) 1732-1738.

[56]   R.M. Glickman and P.H. Green. The intestine as a source of apolipoprotein A1. *Proc. Natl. Acad. Sci. U.S.A.* **74** (1977) 2569-2573.

[57]   A.L. Wu and H.G. Windmueller. Relative contributions by liver and intestine to individual plasma apolipoproteins in the rat. *J. Biol. Chem.* **254** (1979) 7316-7322.

[58]   M. Bodzioch, E. Orso, J. Klucken *et al.* The gene encoding ATP-binding cassette transporter 1 is mutated in Tangier disease. *Nat. Genet.* **22** (1999) 347-351. Comment in: *Nat. Genet.* **22** (1999) 316-318.

[59]   A. Brooks-Wilson, M. Marcil, S.M. Clee *et al.* Mutations in ABC1 in Tangier disease and familial high-density lipoprotein deficiency. *Nat. Genet.* **22** (1999) 336-345. Comment in: *Nat. Genet.* **22** (1999) 316-318.

[60]   S. Rust, M. Rosier, H. Funke *et al.* Tangier disease is caused by mutations in the gene encoding ATP-binding cassette transporter 1. *Nat. Genet.* **22** (1999) 352-355. Comment in: *Nat. Genet.* **22** (1999) 316-318.

[61]   C.L. Wellington, E.K. Walker, A. Suarez *et al.* ABCA1 mRNA and protein distribution patterns predict multiple different roles and levels of regulation. *Lab. Invest.* **82** (2002) 273-283.

[62]   M. Haghpassand, P.A. Bourassa, O.L. Francone *et al.* Monocyte/macrophage expression of ABCA1 has minimal contribution to plasma HDL levels. *J. Clin. Invest.* **108** (2001) 1315-1320. Comment in: *J. Clin. Invest.* **108** (2001) 1273-1275.

[63]   M. van Eck, I.S. Bos, W.E. Kaminski *et al.* Leukocyte ABCA1 controls susceptibility to atherosclerosis and macrophage recruitment into tissues. *Proc. Natl. Acad. Sci. U.S.A.* **99** (2002) 6298-6303.

[64]   M. van Eck, R.R. Singaraja, D. Ye *et al.* Macrophage ATP-binding cassette transporter A1 overexpression inhibits atherosclerotic lesion progression in low-density lipoprotein receptor knockout mice. *Arterioscler. Thromb. Vasc. Biol.* **26** (2006) 929-934.

[65]   F. Basso, L. Freeman, C.L. Knapper *et al.* Role of the hepatic ABCA1 transporter in modulating intrahepatic cholesterol and plasma HDL cholesterol concentrations. *J. Lipid Res.* **44** (2003) 296-302.

[66]   C.L. Wellington, L.R. Brunham, S. Zhou *et al.* Alterations of plasma lipids in mice via adenoviral-mediated hepatic overexpression of human ABCA1. *J. Lipid Res.* **44** (2003) 1470-1480.

[67]   S. Ragozin, A. Niemeier, A. Laatsch *et al.* Knockdown of hepatic ABCA1 by RNA interference decreases plasma HDL cholesterol levels and influences postprandial lipemia in mice. *Arterioscler. Thromb. Vasc. Biol.* **25** (2005) 1433-1438.

[68]   J.M. Timmins, J.Y. Lee, E. Boudyguina *et al.* Targeted inactivation of hepatic Abca1 causes profound hypoalphalipoproteinemia and kidney hypercatabolism of apoA-I. *J. Clin. Invest.* **115** (2005) 1333-1342.

[69]   L.R. Brunham, J.K. Kruit, J. Iqbal *et al.* Intestinal ABCA1 directly contributes to HDL biogenesis in vivo. *J. Clin. Invest.* **116** (2006) 1052-1062.

[70]   S.B. Joseph, E. McKilligin, L. Pei *et al.* Synthetic LXR ligand inhibits the development of atherosclerosis in mice. *Proc. Natl. Acad. Sci. U.S.A.* **99** (2002) 7604-7609.

[71]   N. Terasaka, A. Hiroshima, T. Koieyama *et al.* T-0901317, a synthetic liver X receptor ligand, inhibits development of atherosclerosis in LDL receptor-deficient mice. *FEBS Lett.* **536** (2003) 6-11. Comment in: *FEBS Lett.* **536** (2003) 3-5.

[72]   L.R. Brunham, J.K. Kruit, T.D. Pape *et al.* Tissue-specific induction of intestinal ABCA1 expression with a liver X receptor agonist raises plasma HDL cholesterol levels. *Circ. Res.* **99** (2006) 672-674.

NR4A Nuclear Receptors in the Vessel Wall

Claudia M. van Tiel and Carlie J.M. de Vries
*Department of Medical Biochemistry, Academic Medical Center, University of Amsterdam,
Meibergdreef 15, 1105 AZ Amsterdam, The Netherlands*

Abstract. The NR4A subfamily of nuclear orphan receptors comprises three members Nur77, Nurr1 and NOR-1 that are each expressed in the vessel wall in response to injury and in atherosclerotic lesion macrophages. To study the function of NR4As in vascular smooth muscle cells, endothelial cells and monocyte/macrophages gain of function and siRNA-mediated knock-down experiments have been performed in cultured cells and in dedicated mouse models. Nur77 has been shown to inhibit the formation of smooth muscle cell-rich lesions, to promote endothelial cell survival and to modulate the inflammatory response of macrophages. Most recently, small-molecule activators of NR4As such as 6-mercaptopurine have been identified to modulate the transcriptional activity of these nuclear receptors in experimental model systems. In this chapter we will present the knowledge currently available on vascular actions of NR4As and the function of these nuclear receptors in metabolism will be reviewed briefly. A clinical perspective to approach NR4As as targets for intervention in vascular disease will be given as well as directions for future research.

Keywords. Nuclear orphan receptors, NR4A, vascular biology, atherosclerosis, metabolism

1. Introduction

1.1. General Introduction on Nuclear Receptors

Nuclear receptors (NRs) are ligand-inducible, structurally related transcription factors that regulate the activity of genetic networks in response to a wide variety of signals [1]. They control processes such as cell growth, development and metabolism [2,3]. NRs can be subdivided in three classes. Type I receptors are the classical steroid receptors like the estrogen receptor, the androgen receptor and the glucocorticoid receptor, which upon activation by ligand translocate to the nucleus. Type II receptors are thyroid/retinoid receptors, like the thyroid receptor (TR), the peroxisome proliferator-activated receptors (PPARs) and the retinoic acid receptor (RAR). These receptors are often retained in the nucleus regardless of the presence of their cognate ligands. The last class, class III, comprises the orphan receptors, which were originally identified based on amino-acid sequence similarities with known receptors. However, the ligands of these receptors have not yet been identified. All classes of NRs share a common structural organization. They consist of a highly conserved central DNA-binding domain (DBD), a less conserved carboxy-terminal ligand-binding domain (LDB) and a highly variable amino-terminal transactivation domain [4]. The DBD contains two zinc fingers and is responsible for targeting the receptors to their hormone response elements (HRE). The NRs can bind to DNA as homodimers and/or as heterodimers with Retinoid X Receptor (RXR) with each monomer recognizing a six base pair sequence of DNA, however some NRs can also bind to DNA as monomers. The LBD contains the ligand-binding pocket, which binds small lipophilic ligands such as steroid hormones, retinoids or thyroid hormone, and is responsible for the specificity and selectivity of the physiologic response [4]. The transcriptional activity of NRs is not only regulated by ligand binding, but also modulated by the binding of co-activators, like SRC1/p160, GRIP1/TIF2/SRC2 and CBP/p300, which amplify the transcriptional activity of the NR when recruited, and of co-repressors, which attenuate the activity of the non-activated receptors. It has been shown by X-ray crystallography of several LBDs in the presence or absence of ligand that binding of the ligand induces a conformational change, which results in the loss of interaction with co-repressors and allows co-activators to bind. Many co-activators share a common α-helical LXXLL motif, which can bind to a shallow hydrophobic groove with a charged glutamic and lysine residue lining the rim forming a charged clamp. This surface is exposed after ligand binding due to the conformational change in the LBD of the NR [5,6]. In the absence of ligand the LBD conformation allows co-repressors like NCoR and SMRT to be recruited to NRs. The amino-terminal transactivation domain is important in mediating transcriptional activation. This domain is the least conserved domain between the NRs, both in length and amino-acid composition and has been described to contain the activation function-1 (AF-1) domain.

1.2. Introduction on Members of the NR4A Subfamily of Nuclear Receptors

The NR4A subfamily of nuclear receptors contains three members: Nur77 (NR4A1, TR3, NGFI-B, NAK-1), Nurr1 (NR4A2, NOT) and NOR-1 (NR4A3, MINOR). Nur77 was originally identified in PC12 cells and named NGFI-B, as a factor of which the expression was strongly up-regulated by nerve growth factor [7]. The NR4A subgroup is unique within the large family of NRs by being encoded by immediate early genes that are rapidly and transiently induced by various stimuli. NR4As are expressed in tissues including thymus, muscle, lung, liver, testes, adipose tissue and in the hypothalamus-pituitary-adrenal axis. Although Nur77 knock-out mice do not show an overt phenotype [8], other studies have shown that Nur77 is rapidly induced by T-cell receptor signalling in immature thymocytes and T-cell hybridomas where it plays a role in thymocyte-negative selection and T-cell receptor-mediated apoptosis [9,10]. The involvement of Nur77 in apoptosis is also observed in various cancer cells, like lung, prostate, colon and gastric cancer cells [11-14]. Nurr1 was first detected in brain where it was found to be highly expressed in the dopaminergic neurons of the midbrain [15,16]. Studies using knock-out mice lacking Nurr1 demonstrated that Nurr1 is important for dopamine nerve development as these mice fail to generate these dopaminergic neurons and die soon after birth [17,18]. The third member of the NR4A family was first cloned from cultured rat neuronal cells undergoing apoptosis and was designated as NOR-1 (neuron-derived orphan receptor) [19]. NOR-1 has also been detected as an EWS-NOR-1 fusion protein in myeloid chondrosarcoma, where chromosomal translocation resulted in an EWS chimeric gene encoding a protein in which the amino-terminal transactivation domain of EWS is linked to full-length NOR-1 [20,21]. NOR-1 knock-out mice have been generated in which the NOR-1 gene is disrupted by insertion of *lacZ*. These mice are viable and only have minor problems in inner ear development [22]. However, NOR-1 knock-out mice that were generated by deletion of part of the transactivation domain and the first zinc finger domain show a very different phenotype. The complete absence of NOR-1 protein in the latter mice resulted in embryonic lethality [23].

All three NR4As bind as monomer to an extended HRE (NBRE, AAAGGTCA), or as homodimers to the palindromic NurRE (TGATATTTX6AAAGTCCA) [24]. Nur77 and

Nurr1, but not NOR-1 also form heterodimers with RXR in the presence of retinoids and thus can modulate the activities of a subclass of retinoid REs [25]. Since no physiological ligands for the NR4A receptors have been identified, they belong to the orphan NRs. In fact, crystallographic studies show that the Nurr1 LBD does not contain a ligand-binding pocket, because bulky hydrophobic residues occupy the space that is available for ligand binding, which is different from the LBD of other NRs. Since in the absence of a ligand Nurr1 in the crystal is folded in such a way that it closely resembles the structure of a ligand-bound, transcriptionally active LBD of other NRs, it is thought that the transcriptional activity of the NR4A receptors is independent of ligands. In addition, NR4A receptors lack the classical hydrophobic co-activator binding groove, where in other NRs LXXLL-containing proteins can bind. In Nurr1 this groove is filled with polar side chains [26]. Recently a new co-regulator binding surface has been identified in the Nurr1 LBD which was shown to bind non-polar peptides derived from the co-repressors NCoR and SMRT [27,28]. The function of this surface in regulation of NR4A activity needs, however, to be assessed in more detail. Although as yet there are no endogenous ligands known for the NR4A receptors, recently several compounds that activate NR4As *in vitro* have been identified. It has been shown that the antineoplastic and anti-inflammatory drug 6-mercaptopurine (6-MP) increases NR4A transactivation via its N-terminal transactivation domain. The exact mechanism by which 6-MP enhances the transcriptional activity of the NR4A receptors is unknown, however, it has been shown that the activation does not involve direct interaction between 6-MP and the receptor [29,30]. Recently a series of methylene-substituted diindolylmethanes (DIM-Cs) were identified as Nur77 agonists. Interestingly, these DIM-Cs activate Nur77 through its LBD and binding of Nur77 to its RE is not affected [31]. Whether this effect on transactivation involves direct binding of DIM-Cs to the LBD remains to be elucidated.

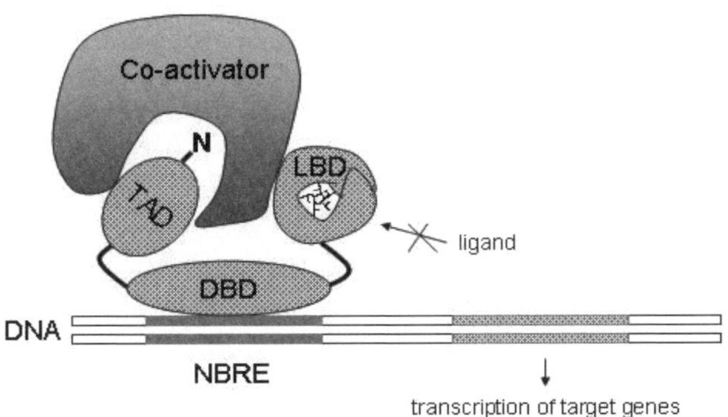

Figure 1. Schematic representation of the structure of NR4A nuclear receptors.

2. NR4A Nuclear Receptors in Metabolism

One of the major risk factors for atherosclerosis is obesity, which leads to elevated triglyceride and low-density lipoprotein (bad) cholesterol levels, impaired fasting glucose and hypertension. Liver, adipose tissue and skeletal muscle are crucial tissues in basal metabolism and have significant roles in blood-lipid and glucose profiles and energy homeostasis. Both Nur77 and NOR-1 are strongly induced in skeletal muscle in response to β-adrenergic stimulation and siRNA knock-down studies revealed that Nur77 and NOR-1 promote lipolysis in this tissue [32,33]. All three NR4A subfamily members are expressed in mice after cold exposure in brown adipose tissue and in fasting liver when glucagon levels are increased. Nur77 has been shown to induce the expression of glucose-6-phosphate phosphatase, fructose-1,6-biphosphate phosphatase-1 and -2 and enolase 3 in liver cells and to increase fasting glucose levels in mice after over-expression in the liver [34]. Inactivation of NR4A activity by means of over-expression of a dominant-negative variant in the liver inhibits the expression of gluconeogenic genes and lowers blood glucose levels in diabetic mice [34].

3. NR4A Nuclear Receptors in the Vessel Wall

Atherosclerosis is a disease of the arteries with a focal appearance, in which areas of the vascular tree with relatively low shear stress, such as occurs at curves and bifurcations, are prone to develop vascular lesions in response to systemic factors. At these specific sites the endothelium, which lines the vessel lumen, becomes activated allowing circulating monocytes to bind and extravasate into the vascular wall. Local accumulation of reactive oxygen species and oxidized lipoproteins activate the infiltrated macrophages resulting in the release of excessive cytokines and chemokines attracting even more inflammatory cells (macrophages and T-cells). Also medial smooth muscle cells (SMCs) become activated and migrate and proliferate into the lesion area. Macrophages scavenge (modified) lipids and become large so-called foam-cells that become physically trapped in the vessel wall. Eventually, complex atherosclerotic lesions are formed that gradually obstruct normal blood flow, but these lesions can also in an earlier stage of the disease rupture and cause local blood coagulation resulting in an acute ischemic event. In addition to atherosclerotic lesions, also SMC-rich lesions may be formed in the vessel wall. For example, after stent placement in angioplastic procedures, accelerated restenotic lesions can develop, which are composed predominantly of SMCs. Similarly, in vein-graft disease, a complication of venous bypass-grafting, vascular lesions are formed that are rich in proliferating SMCs.

NR4A nuclear receptors are expressed under specific conditions in vascular SMCs, endothelial cells, T-cells and macrophages. Each of these cell-types is involved in vascular lesion formation, and in this chapter we present the data currently available on cellular functions that are affected by Nur77, Nurr1 and/or NOR-1 in these specific cell-types (Figure 2).

3.1. NR4As in Vascular Smooth Muscle Cells

In SMCs Nur77 and Nurr1 were originally identified as genes that are expressed upon activation of human cells by differential display analysis, whereas NOR-1 was recognized in porcine SMCs by the same technique [35,36]. NR4A factors show in SMCs a transient and immediate early expression pattern in response to diverse stimuli, such as serum, low-density lipoprotein (LDL), platelet-derived growth factor (PDGF) and mechanical strain. It has now been shown extensively that induction of NOR-1 gene expression involves cAMP-response element binding protein (CREB) and CREB-response elements in the NOR-1 promoter in SMCs, similar as in breast cancer cells [36-39]. We have shown that all three NR4As are expressed in human atherosclerotic lesions but not in medial SMCs of the normal, quiescent vessel wall [40]. Furthermore, we observed expression of Nur77 in human saphenous vein segments exposed *ex vivo* to whole-blood perfusion under arterial pressure and in cultured venous SMCs challenged by cyclic stretch, to mimic excessive mechanical strain on venous SMCs *in vitro* [41]. Nur77 expression has also been observed in lesions that develop after placement of a loosely-fitting cuff around the mouse femoral artery [42] and NOR-1 expression is induced in porcine coronary arteries in response to percutaneous transluminal coronary angioplasty-mediated injury [36].

To delineate the function of NR4As in SMCs gain and loss-of-function experiments have been performed. It has been proposed that NOR-1 promotes SMC proliferation and migration, since antisense oligonucleotides directed against NOR-1 mRNA inhibit serum- and LDL-induced growth of vascular SMCs, as well as migration of SMCs in a scratch-wound assay [36,38]. These data were further substantiated by experiments with primary murine SMCs that were derived from NOR-1 knock-out animals [22]; wild-type littermate SMCs showed a selective growth advantage relative to NOR-1-deficient SMCs, both in response to serum and in response to PDGF. Growth inhibition of these NOR-1-deficient SMCs was rescued by re-introduction of NOR-1 cDNA [39]. It should be noted, however, that these NOR-1 knock-out mice are viable and were shown to develop only a minor ear defect, whereas the NOR-1 knock-out mice generated by Winoto and coworkers exhibit an early embryonic lethal phenotype [23].

Venous SMCs, in contrast to mammary artery-derived SMCs, proliferate in response to cyclic stretch. To reveal the growth inhibitory function of Nur77 in stretch-activation of SMCs, we have demonstrated that siRNA-mediated knock-down of Nur77 and over-expression of Nur77 in venous SMCs result in enhanced and abolished stretch-induced DNA synthesis, respectively. Moreover, stretch-mediated SMC proliferation was shown to be inhibited by 6-MP, in a Nur77-dependent way. To study the function of Nur77 in SMC-rich lesion formation *in vivo* we generated transgenic mice over-expressing Nur77 under control of the SM22α-promoter, which directs transgene expression to arterial SMCs [43,44]. The mice were challenged by carotid artery ligation and it was demonstrated that SMC-rich lesion formation was reduced in Nur77-over-expressing mice [40]. To evaluate the contribution of endogenous NR4A factors in the formation of such lesions, we applied a well-described dominant-negative variant of Nur77, denoted Nur77-ΔTA, which lacks the amino-terminal transactivation domain and inhibits the transcriptional activity of all three NR4As [45]. Nur77-ΔTA transgenic mice (with the same SM22α-promoter) were generated and these mice develop more lesion than their wild-type littermates indicating that inhibition of all three NR4A subfamily members in the vessel wall aggravates lesion formation [40]. To further explore the function of Nur77 in SMC-rich lesion formation and to answer the question whether Nur77 may be targeted with its small-molecule activators, we applied 6-MP in a mouse model with drug-eluting cuffs and showed that locally applied 6-MP indeed inhibits lesion formation. Moreover, in transgenic mice over-expressing Nur77 in the vessel wall we observed a stronger inhibition, whereas lesion formation was no longer influenced by local 6-MP application when the dominant-negative variant Nur77-ΔTA is present in the vessel wall [42].

Based on these data we concluded that Nur77 protects against the formation of SMC-rich lesion formation, which is of special interest because Nur77 is only expressed in vascular lesions and not in the normal vessel wall. Consequently, we propose that Nur77 is involved in endogenous feedback mechanisms that are set off upon activation of SMCs to modulate excessive cellular proliferation.

3.2. NR4As in Endothelial Cells

In cultured vascular endothelial cells, NR4A expression is transiently and robustly induced by serum and vascular endothelial growth factor (VEGF) [46,47]. For Nur77 it has been shown that its transcription is directly regulated by hypoxia-inducible factor-1 (HIF-1α) in hypoxic renal cell carcinoma [48] and that Nur77 in turn stabilizes HIF-1α [49]. Based on gain of function experiments for Nur77 we proposed that Nur77 inhibits cell-cycle progression and may be involved in maintenance of vascular endothelium integrity [46], whereas antisense oligonucleotide-mediated knock-down of NOR-1 has been shown to inhibit endothelial cell proliferation, indicating that NOR-1 promotes the growth of these cells. In a mouse angiogenesis model [50] it has been demonstrated that VEGF-mediated angiogenesis is dependent on Nur77 expression and transcriptional activity. Most recently, it has been shown that 6-MP enhances the expression of all three NR4A members and promotes endothelial cell tube formation [51]. Together, these data may indicate that NR4As promote endothelial cell survival and are involved in angiogenesis.

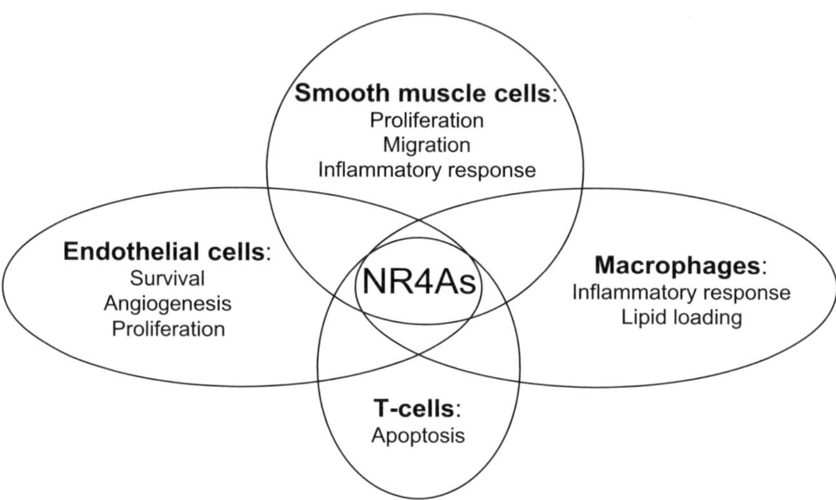

Figure 2. Schematic representation of the cells involved in initiation and progression of vascular disease and specific cellular functions modulated by NR4A nuclear receptors.

3.3. NR4As in T-cells and Macrophages

As indicated in the introduction, atherosclerosis is a chronic inflammatory disease involving the action of T-cells and macrophages in the vessel wall both at the initiation and during progression of vascular disease. Winoto and coworkers performed extensive studies on the function of NR4As in (developing) T-cells and demonstrated that both Nur77 and NOR-1 induce apoptosis in T-cells [52]. Subsequent studies, involving microarray analyses, revealed that Nur77 induces apoptosis through transcriptional activation of many genes, including known apoptotic genes such as FasL and TRAIL [53]. Also in macrophages Nur77 has been implicated to be involved in apoptosis, however, this study shows that only in the presence of zVAD (a pan-caspase inhibitor) Nur77 induces caspase-independent apoptosis in these cells. In human and mouse monocytes and macrophages all three NR4A factors are robustly, rapidly and transiently induced upon activation of these cells by phorbol-esters, LPS, cytokines such as TNFα and by oxidized LDL [54,55]. Pei *et al* have shown that the induction of expression of Nur77 in macrophages in response to inflammatory signals involves NFκB-activity, which subsequently results in enhanced expression of multiple genes among which IKKi/IKKε, a modulator of the NFκB signalling cascade, and TNFα and IP10/CXCL10 [54,56]. We demonstrated that over-expression of each of the NR4A factors in monocytic THP-1 cells, results in reduced expression of the pro-inflammatory cytokines interleukin (IL)-1β and IL-6 and the chemokines IL-8, macrophage inflammatory protein (MIP)-1α and -1β and monocyte chemoattractant protein-1 (MCP1) in THP-1 derived macrophages. In addition, NR4A-factors reduce oxidized-low-density lipoprotein uptake, consistent with down-regulation of scavenger receptor-A, CD36, and CD11b macrophage marker genes. Knock-down of Nur77 or NOR-1 with gene-specific lentiviral short-hairpin RNAs resulted in enhanced cytokine and chemokine synthesis, increased lipid loading, and augmented CD11b expression, demonstrating endogenous NR4A-factors to indeed inhibit macrophage activation, foam-cell formation, and differentiation. Based on these results we hypothesized that NR4As have an anti-inflammatory function in macrophages and are protective in vascular lesion formation. So far, however, no *in vivo* data are available on functional involvement of NR4A factors in T-cell and macrophage function in atherosclerotic lesions.

4. Future Directions and Clinical Perspectives for NR4A Nuclear Receptors

The NR4A nuclear receptors Nur77, Nurr1 and NOR-1 are expressed upon activation of specific cells crucial in basal metabolism and vascular lesion formation as reviewed in this chapter. At present, relatively little is known on the genes that are regulated downstream of these transcription factors, therefore gene expression profiling experiments in vascular cells are warranted. NR4A nuclear receptors comprise unique structures in their ligand-binding domains, which may exclude binding of traditional ligands, and the presence of a novel molecule surface is predicted to interact with (novel) co-activator and co-repressor proteins. Again, only limited knowledge is available on NR4A-interacting proteins, both at the C-terminal and at the N-terminal (AF-1) domain, which may be subject of future studies to reveal the exact mechanism of action of NR4As. Based on the knowledge that Nur77 promotes endothelial cell survival, inhibits SMC proliferation, enhances T-cell apoptosis, and reduces the uptake of modified lipoproteins and the inflammatory response of macrophages, we propose that Nur77 is protective in vascular disease. Modulating the activity of NR4A nuclear receptors with small-molecule activators, such as 6-MP or DIM-Cs, may therefore be considered as a rational objective to locally treat vascular lesion formation.

References

[1]   N.J. McKenna and B.W. O'Malley. Combinatorial control of gene expression by nuclear receptors and coregulators. *Cell* **108** (2002) 465-474.

[2]   D.L. Bain, A.F. Heneghan, K.D. Connaghan-Jones *et al.* Nuclear receptor structure: implications for function. *Annu. Rev. Physiol* **69** (2007) 201-220.

[3]   R.C. Ribeiro, P.J. Kushner, J.D. Baxter. The nuclear hormone receptor gene superfamily. *Annu. Rev. Med.* **46** (1995) 443-453.

[4]   D.J. Mangelsdorf, C. Thummel, M. Beato *et al.* The nuclear receptor superfamily: the second decade. *Cell* **83** (1995) 835-839.

[5]   D.M. Heery, E. Kalkhoven, S. Hoare *et al.* A signature motif in transcriptional co-activators mediates binding to nuclear receptors. *Nature* **387** (1997) 733-736. Comment in: *Nature* **387** (1997) 654-655.

[6]   B.D. Darimont, R.L. Wagner, J.W. Apriletti *et al.* Structure and specificity of nuclear receptor-coactivator interactions. *Genes Dev.* **12** (1998) 3343-3356.

[7]   J. Milbrandt. Nerve growth factor induces a gene homologous to the glucocorticoid receptor gene. *Neuron* **1** (1988) 183-188.

[8]   S.L. Lee, R.L. Wesselschmidt, G.P. Linette *et al.* Unimpaired thymic and peripheral T cell death in mice lacking the nuclear receptor NGFI-B (Nur77). *Science* **269** (1995) 532-535.

[9]   Z.G. Liu, S.W. Smith, K.A. McLaughlin *et al.* Apoptotic signals delivered through the T-cell receptor of a T-cell hybrid require the immediate-early gene nur77. *Nature* **367** (1994) 281-284.

[10]   J.D. Woronicz, B. Calnan, V. Ngo *et al.* Requirement for the orphan steroid receptor Nur77 in apoptosis of T-cell hybridomas. *Nature* **367** (1994) 277-281.

[11]   Y. Li, B. Lin, A. Agadir *et al.* Molecular determinants of AHPN (CD437)-induced growth arrest and apoptosis in human lung cancer cell lines. *Mol. Cell. Biol.* **18** (1998) 4719-4731.

[12]   H. Uemura and C. Chang. Antisense TR3 orphan receptor can increase prostate cancer cell viability with etoposide treatment. *Endocrinology* **139** (1998) 2329-2334.

[13]   A.J. Wilson, D. Arango, J.M. Mariadason *et al.* TR3/Nur77 in colon cancer cell apoptosis. *Cancer Res.* **63** (2003) 5401-5407.

[14]   Q. Wu, S. Liu, X.F. Ye *et al.* Dual roles of Nur77 in selective regulation of apoptosis and cell cycle by TPA and ATRA in gastric cancer cells. *Carcinogenesis* **23** (2002) 1583-1592.

[15]   S.W. Law, O.M. Conneely, F.J. DeMayo *et al.* Identification of a new brain-specific transcription factor, NURR1. *Mol. Endocrinol.* **6** (1992) 2129-2135.

[16]   R.H. Zetterstrom, R. Williams, T. Perlmann *et al.* Cellular expression of the immediate early transcription factors Nurr1 and NGFI-B suggests a gene regulatory role in several brain regions including the nigrostriatal dopamine system. *Brain Res. Mol. Brain Res.* **41** (1996) 111-120.

[17]   R.H. Zetterstrom, L. Solomin, L. Jansson *et al.* Dopamine neuron agenesis in Nurr1-deficient mice. *Science* **276** (1997) 248-250. Comment in: *Science* **276** (1997) 202.

[18]   O. Saucedo-Cardenas, J.D. Quintana-Hau, W.D. Le *et al.* Nurr1 is essential for the induction of the dopaminergic phenotype and the survival of ventral mesencephalic late dopaminergic precursor neurons. *Proc. Natl. Acad. Sci. U.S.A.* **95** (1998) 4013-4018.

[19]   N. Ohkura, M. Hijikuro, A. Yamamoto *et al.* Molecular cloning of a novel thyroid/steroid receptor superfamily gene from cultured rat neuronal cells. *Biochem. Biophys. Res. Commun.* **205** (1994) 1959-1965.

[20]   Y. Labelle, J. Zucman, G. Stenman *et al.* Oncogenic conversion of a novel orphan nuclear receptor by chromosome translocation. *Hum. Mol. Genet.* **4** (1995) 2219-2226.

[21]   J. Clark, H. Benjamin, S. Gill *et al.* Fusion of the EWS gene to CHN, a member of the steroid/thyroid receptor gene superfamily, in a human myxoid chondrosarcoma. *Oncogene* **12** (1996) 229-235.

[22]   T. Ponnio, Q. Burton, F.A. Pereira *et al.* The nuclear receptor Nor-1 is essential for proliferation of the semicircular canals of the mouse inner ear. *Mol. Cell. Biol.* **22** (2002) 935-945.

[23]   R.A. DeYoung, J.C. Baker, D. Cado *et al.* The orphan steroid receptor Nur77 family member Nor-1 is essential for early mouse embryogenesis. *J. Biol. Chem.* **278** (2003) 47104-47109.

[24]   A. Philips, S. Lesage, R. Gingras *et al.* Novel dimeric Nur77 signaling mechanism in endocrine and lymphoid cells. *Mol. Cell. Biol.* **17** (1997) 5946-5951.

[25]   T. Perlmann and L. Jansson. A novel pathway for vitamin A signaling mediated by RXR heterodimerization with NGFI-B and NURR1. *Genes Dev.* **9** (1995) 769-782.

[26]   Z. Wang, G. Benoit, J. Liu *et al.* Structure and function of Nurr1 identifies a class of ligand-independent nuclear receptors. *Nature* **423** (2003) 555-560.

[27]   N. Volakakis, M. Malewicz, B. Kadkhodai *et al.* Characterization of the Nurr1 ligand-binding domain co-activator interaction surface. *J. Mol. Endocrinol.* **37** (2006) 317-326.

[28]   A. Codina, G. Benoit, J.T. Gooch *et al.* Identification of a novel co-regulator interaction surface on the ligand binding domain of Nurr1 using NMR footprinting. *J. Biol. Chem.* **279** (2004) 53338-53345.

[29]   P. Ordentlich, Y. Yan, S. Zhou *et al.* Identification of the antineoplastic agent 6-mercaptopurine as an activator of the orphan nuclear hormone receptor Nurr1. *J. Biol. Chem.* **278** (2003) 24791-24799.

[30]   K.D. Wansa, J.M. Harris, G. Yan *et al.* The AF-1 domain of the orphan nuclear receptor NOR-1 mediates trans-activation, coactivator recruitment, and activation by the purine anti-metabolite 6-mercaptopurine. *J. Biol. Chem.* **278** (2003) 24776-24790.

[31]   S. Chintharlapalli, R. Burghardt, S. Papineni *et al.* Activation of Nur77 by selected 1,1-Bis(3'-indolyl)-1-(p-substituted phenyl)methanes induces apoptosis through nuclear pathways. *J. Biol. Chem.* **280** (2005) 24903-24914.

[32]   M.A. Maxwell, M.E. Cleasby, A. Harding *et al.* Nur77 regulates lipolysis in skeletal muscle cells. Evidence for cross-talk between the beta-adrenergic and an orphan nuclear hormone receptor pathway. *J. Biol. Chem.* **280** (2005) 12573-12584.

[33]   M.A. Pearen, J.G. Ryall, M.A. Maxwell *et al.* The orphan nuclear receptor, NOR-1, is a target of beta-adrenergic signaling in skeletal muscle. *Endocrinology* **147** (2006) 5217-5227.

[34]   L. Pei, H. Waki, B. Vaitheesvaran *et al.* NR4A orphan nuclear receptors are transcriptional regulators of hepatic glucose metabolism. *Nat. Med.* **12** (2006) 1048-1055.

[35]   C.J. de Vries, T.A. van Achterberg, A.J. Horrevoets *et al.* Differential display identification of 40 genes with altered expression in activated human smooth muscle cells. Local expression in atherosclerotic lesions of smags, smooth muscle activation-specific genes. *J. Biol. Chem.* **275** (2000) 23939-23947.

[36]　J. Martinez-Gonzalez, J. Rius, A. Castello *et al.* Neuron-derived orphan receptor-1 (NOR-1) modulates vascular smooth muscle cell proliferation. *Circ. Res.* **92** (2003) 96-103.

[37]　T. Ohkubo, N. Ohkura, K. Maruyama *et al.* Early induction of the orphan nuclear receptor NOR-1 during cell death of the human breast cancer cell line MCF-7. *Mol. Cell. Endocrinol.* **162** (2000) 151-156.

[38]　J. Rius, J. Martinez-Gonzalez, J. Crespo *et al.* Involvement of neuron-derived orphan receptor-1 (NOR-1) in LDL-induced mitogenic stimulus in vascular smooth muscle cells: role of CREB. *Arterioscler. Thromb. Vasc. Biol.* **24** (2004) 697-702.

[39]　T. Nomiyama, T. Nakamachi, F. Gizard *et al.* The NR4A orphan nuclear receptor NOR1 is induced by platelet-derived growth factor and mediates vascular smooth muscle cell proliferation. *J. Biol. Chem.* **281** (2006) 33467-33476.

[40]　E.K. Arkenbout, V. de Waard, M. van Bragt *et al.* Protective function of transcription factor TR3 orphan receptor in atherogenesis: decreased lesion formation in carotid artery ligation model in TR3 transgenic mice. *Circulation* **106** (2002) 1530-1535.

[41]　V. de Waard, E.K. Arkenbout, M. Vos *et al.* TR3 nuclear orphan receptor prevents cyclic stretch-induced proliferation of venous smooth muscle cells. *Am. J. Pathol.* **168** (2006) 2027-2035.

[42]　N.M. Pires, T.W. Pols, M.R. de Vries *et al.* Activation of nuclear receptor Nur77 by 6-mercaptopurine protects against neointima formation. *Circulation* **115** (2007) 493-500.

[43]　J. Solway, J. Seltzer, F.F. Samaha *et al.* Structure and expression of a smooth muscle cell-specific gene, SM22 alpha. *J. Biol. Chem.* **270** (1995) 13460-13469.

[44]　L. Li, J.M. Miano, B. Mercer *et al.* Expression of the SM22alpha promoter in transgenic mice provides evidence for distinct transcriptional regulatory programs in vascular and visceral smooth muscle cells. *J. Cell Biol.* **132** (1996) 849-859.

[45]　B.J. Calnan, S. Szychowski, F.K. Chan *et al.* A role for the orphan steroid receptor Nur77 in apoptosis accompanying antigen-induced negative selection. *Immunity* **3** (1995) 273-282.

[46]　E.K. Arkenbout, M. van Bragt, E. Eldering *et al.* TR3 orphan receptor is expressed in vascular endothelial cells and mediates cell cycle arrest. *Arterioscler. Thromb. Vasc. Biol.* **23** (2003) 1535-1540.

[47]　D. Liu, H. Jia, D.I. Holmes *et al.* Vascular endothelial growth factor-regulated gene expression in endothelial cells: KDR-mediated induction of Egr3 and the related nuclear receptors Nur77, Nurr1, and Nor1. *Arterioscler. Thromb. Vasc. Biol.* **23** (2003) 2002-2007.

[48]　J.W. Choi, S.C. Park, G.H. Kang *et al.* Nur77 activated by hypoxia-inducible factor-1alpha overproduces proopiomelanocortin in von Hippel-Lindau-mutated renal cell carcinoma. *Cancer Res.* **64** (2004) 35-39.

[49]　Y.G. Yoo, M.G. Yeo, D.K. Kim *et al.* Novel function of orphan nuclear receptor Nur77 in stabilizing hypoxia-inducible factor-1alpha. *J. Biol. Chem.* **279** (2004) 53365-53373.

[50]　H. Zeng, L. Qin, D. Zhao *et al.* Orphan nuclear receptor TR3/Nur77 regulates VEGF-A-induced angiogenesis through its transcriptional activity. *J. Exp. Med.* **203** (2006) 719-729.

[51]　Y.G. Yoo, T.Y. Na, W.K. Yang *et al.* 6-Mercaptopurine, an activator of Nur77, enhances transcriptional activity of HIF-1alpha resulting in new vessel formation. *Oncogene* **26** (2007) 3823-3834.

[52]　A. Winoto and D.R. Littman. Nuclear hormone receptors in T lymphocytes. *Cell* **109 Suppl.** (2002) S57-S66.

[53]　A. Rajpal, Y.A. Cho, B. Yelent *et al.* Transcriptional activation of known and novel apoptotic pathways by Nur77 orphan steroid receptor. *EMBO J.* **22** (2003) 6526-6536.

[54]　L. Pei, A. Castrillo, M. Chen *et al.* Induction of NR4A orphan nuclear receptor expression in macrophages in response to inflammatory stimuli. *J. Biol. Chem.* **280** (2005) 29256-29262.

[55]　P.I. Bonta, C.M. van Tiel, M. Vos *et al.* Nuclear receptors Nur77, Nurr1, and NOR-1 expressed in atherosclerotic lesion macrophages reduce lipid loading and inflammatory responses. *Arterioscler. Thromb. Vasc. Biol.* **26** (2006) 2288-2294.

[56]　L. Pei, A. Castrillo, P. Tontonoz. Regulation of macrophage inflammatory gene expression by the orphan nuclear receptor Nur77. *Mol. Endocrinol.* **20** (2006) 786-794.

Nuclear Receptors as Molecular Targets for Cardiometabolic and Central Nervous System Diseases   85
J.L. Junien and B. Staels (Eds.)
IOS Press, 2008

Cholesterol: Novel Target in the Treatment of Alzheimer's Disease?

M. Mulder

Department of Basic Neurosciences, Institute Brain & Behavior, EURON,
Maastricht University, Universiteitssingel 50, 6229 ER Maastricht, The Netherlands

Abstract. At present there are about 250.000 patients with dementia in the Netherlands. Sixty to 70% of these are diagnosed as patients with Alzheimer's disease (AD). Considering the relative increase in the number of elderly people the prevalence of AD will only increase further.

One hundred years after the first description of AD the underlying molecular mechanisms that finally result in the loss of higher cognitive functions still remain to be clarified. At present there is no cure.

Accumulating evidence indicates a link between an aberrant brain cholesterol metabolism and AD. Therefore, modulation of cerebral cholesterol metabolism may be a possible novel strategy in the treatment of the disease. In the present paper the role of cholesterol in AD and the possibilities to use it as a target for treatment will be addressed.

Keywords. Alzheimer's disease, cholesterol metabolism, apolipoprotein E

The german neurologist Aloïs Alzheimer in November 1906 first described the presence of two characteristic neuropathological hallmarks in the brain of his first Alzheimer patient after she died. These were so-called senile plaques, with amyloid-beta as the key protein, and neurofibrillary tangles which are intraneuronal aggregates of an abnormal for of the protein tau (Figure 1). Even now post-mortem the number of plaques and tangles in the hippocampus is being used for the final diagnoses. However, some controversy remains with respect to the contribution of both plaques and tangles to the progressive loss of cognitive functions.

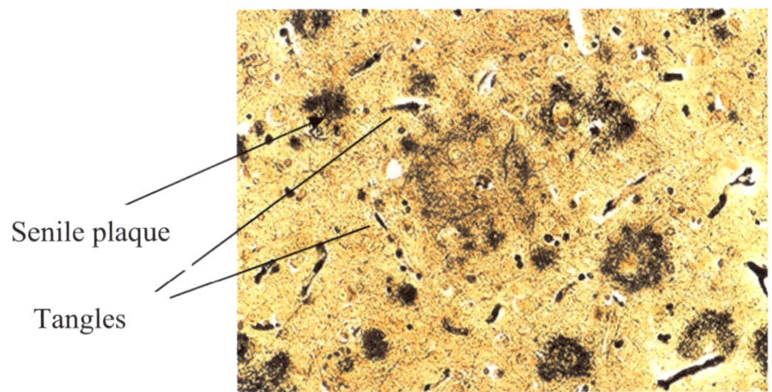

Figure 1. Senile plaques and fibrillary tangles in the brain of an Alzheimer patient.

A strictly regulated brain cholesterol metabolism is required for optimal brain functioning. Disturbances herein can lead to severe neurological diseases such as Smith-Lemli-Opitz syndrome [1], Niemann-Pick type C1 [2] and Cerebrotendinous Xantomatosis [3]. Recently accumulated evidence indicates an important role for an aberrant brain cholesterol metabolism in the development and progression of AD [4,5].

The brain contains about 25% of all free cholesterol of the whole body, while they only represent 2% of the total body weight. All cholesterol within the brain is synthesized locally. The blood-brain barrier (BBB) prevents cholesterol from the circulation from entering the brain [6]. In the brain cholesterol is predominantly present in membranes of myelin and in neuronal and glial membranes, and in contrast with what was generally assumed, it is constantly being replaced. There is a daily turnover of at least 6 mg cholesterol, which is about 1% of the turnover in the rest of the body. Although, the turnover of cholesterol in myelin membranes can be upto 3 years, in a subset of neurons it can be as fast as in the rest of the body. Since cholesterol, in contrast with other lipids, cannot be degraded in the human body, the excess cholesterol is being secreted from the brain in the blood and finally via the liver is being released from the body [7]. About 60% is being secreted in the form of the more polar cholesterol metabolite ^{24}S-hydroxycholesterol (Figure 2) [8,9]. The other 40% is being secreted via another, yet unknown route which may involve apolipoprotein E (ApoE). High concentrations of free cholesterol can lead to the formation of crystals which are toxic to cells and to neurons in particular [10,11]. Also oxysterols, such as ^{24}S-hydroxycholesterol, can be toxic for neurons.

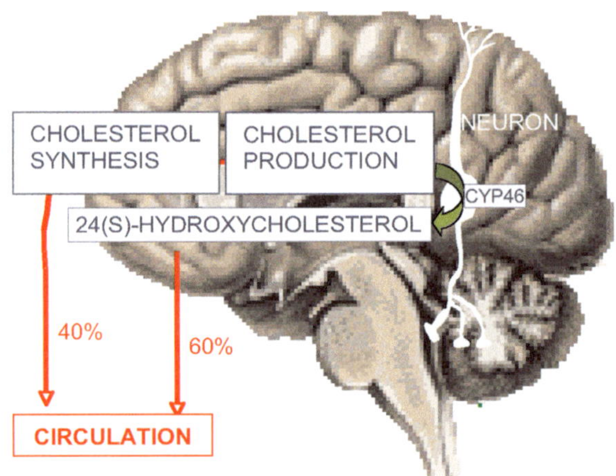

Figure 2. Schematic representation of the cholesterol-turnover in the brain. All cholesterol is being synthesized endogenously and is being secreted in the form of ^{24}S-hydroxycholesterol or via an alternative, yet unknown, pathway

In 1993 the first indication pointing at a link between cholesterol and AD was found. ApoE4, one of the three common forms of ApoE (E2, E3 and E4) was found to be associated with an increased risk of developing AD [12,13]. ApoE is known predominantly because of its role as a cholesterol transporter in the circulation [14]. Also within the brain ApoE is thought to play an important role in the distribution of cholesterol and in the transport of lipids across the BBB [15,16].

The second indication for a link between cholesterol and AD came from epidemiological studies. It was found that the use of cholesterol-lowering drugs, so-called statins that are being used in the treatment of cardiovascular diseases, reduced the risk of AD [17]. Statins were found to reduce the deposition of amyloid-beta in plaques in the brain of AD-mouse-models [18]. These effects were ascribed to the cholesterol-lowering effect of statins. In agreement high plasma cholesterol levels and high-fat intake were found to be associated with an increased risk of AD [19]. Already 10 years ago Sparks *et al* discovered plaques-like structures in brains of patients that died of cardiovascular diseases and not in brain of patients with other causes of death [20]. High plasma cholesterol concentrations results in an increased depositon of amyloid-beta in the brains of AD-mouse-models [21,22]. Cholesterol itself was found to be present in plaques [23].

On the one hand disturbances in cholesterol metabolism appear to affect the development and the progression of AD, but on the other hand a number of studies suggest that alterations in cholesterol metabolism may be the result of the disease. Cerebrospinal fluid of AD patients contains lower concentrations of cholesterol, phospholipids and fatty acids and higher concentrations of ^{24}S-hydroxycholesterol [7,24-28]. A polymorphism in the gene for ^{24}S-hydroxylase (CYP46), that converts cholesterol into ^{24}S-hydroxycholesterol, was found to be associated with AD [29]. Moreover, the distribution of this enzyme in AD brains differed from that in brains from non-demented patients. The observation of an altered processing of cholesterol in fibroblasts from AD patients, suggest that the changes do not remain restricted to the central nervous system [30].

It is not simply the level of cholesterol in the brain that affects the production and deposition of amyloid-beta, but more its intracellular distribution. *In vitro* studies show that the cellular amount of cholesterol or the distribution across membranes directly affects the splicing of amyloid from its precursor protein and on its aggregation [31-33]. Cholesterol-depleted neurons produce less amyloid than cholesterol-rich neurons.

Therefore, alterations in brain cholesterol metabolism seem to affect the production and deposition of amyloid. Alternatively, amyloid-beta also seems to directly affect cholesterol synthesis [34]. The regulation of cholesterol metabolism in the periphery and disturbances herein, have been investigated extensively. However, far less is known with respect to the regulation of cholesterol in the brain, and in particular the alterations that occur during aging or during the progression of AD.

As mentioned before, cholesterol metabolism in the brain is considered to be autonomous. In line with this assumption we found that several-fold increased plasma levels of cholesterol, its precursors and metabolites in ApoE-deficient mice, did not result in any detectable alterations in levels of these sterols in the brain. Even after further increase of plasma sterol levels by administration of a high-fat diet, did not result in any changes in brain sterol levels (unpublished results). However, it did result in severe neuropathology in ApoE-deficient mice but not in wild-type control mice [16].

Recently, we reported that alterations in serum sterol profiles induced via the diet, can be accompanied by alterations in brain sterol profile. We found that increased plant sterol levels in the circulation can lead to increased levels of these sterols in the brain [35]. Plant sterols are retrieved from plants and can therefore only be retrieved from the diet. Since plant sterols have a structure very similar to that of cholesterol, up to recently it was assumed that similar to cholesterol they could not cross the BBB.

Neurons reduce their cholesterol production after birth and subsequently astrocytes provide them with cholesterol. Astrocytes secrete cholesterol associated with ApoE in the form of High-Density-Lipoprotein-like particles, which are being internalized by neurons via up to now largely unknown receptors [36-38]. It is thought that these particles deliver cholesterol to neurons for the formation of new membranes during regeneration after injury or during the formation of synaptic contacts which occurs during a process called synaptic plasticity. Synaptic plasticity is the reorganization of synaptic contacts, a process that occurs in particular in the hippocampus, a brain region involved in learning and memory, which is also one of the first to be affected during the progression of AD.

We wondered how neurons communicate with astrocytes in order to let them now that they need cholesterol. In the human brain [24]S-hydroxycholesterol is specifically formed in neurons [39]. [24]S-hydroxycholesterol is a natural ligand for the Liver X Receptors (LXRs), so-called master regulators of cellular cholesterol homeostasis [40,41]. LXRs belong to the nuclear hormone receptor superfamily. Two forms LXRalpha and LXRbeta have been identified. Both are present in the brain and are thought to be involved in the regulation of brain cholesterol homeostasis [42]. This is supported by the observation that LXRalpha/beta-deficient mice display several defects in their central nervous system. These include closed ventricles, lipid accumulation in astrocytes and around blood vessels, proliferation of astrocytes and dysorganisation of myelin sheaths [43].

Our recent data show that in the brain [24]S-hydroxycholesterol that is derived from neurons, signals to astrocytes and induces the secretion of ApoE-containing lipoprotein-like particles via the LXR-pathway, in order to supply neurons with cholesterol required for regeneration or for the formation of new synapses (Figure 3) [44].

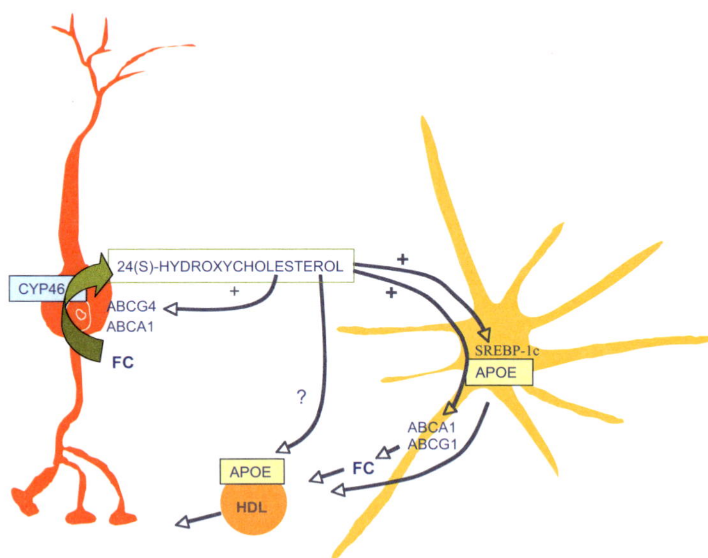

Figure 3. Schematic representation of cell-type specific effects of LXR-activation by [24]S-hydroxycholesterol in astrocytes and neurons on the expression of LXR-target genes including ApoE and ATP-binding cassette (ABC) transporters, as well as on cholesterol efflux.

Alterations in these processes may be involved in the development and the progression of AD, and also in other neurodegenerative diseases.

Since disturbances in cerebral cholesterol metabolism may play an important role in the progression of AD, modulation of hereof may be a possible novel strategy in the treatment of the disease. Potential candidates include "statins" and pharmaceuticals that interfere with the LXR-pathway.

High doses of simvastatin were found to reduce cholesterol synthesis in the brain [45]. Therefore, it was initially suggested that the beneficial effects of statins on the developent of AD may be the result of its cholesterol-lowering effects [46]. However, it is questionable if this is an advantage. The use of statins has also been associated with memory complaints [47]. Furthermore, it was found that statins directly inhibit long-term potentiation, which is regarded as a marker for synaptic plasticity a process required for learning and memory processes [48]. In line Kotti *et al* reported that cholesterol synthesis in the brain is essential for learning processes. It is not cholesterol itself that is required but a non-sterol by-product, the isoprenoid "geranylgeraniol" that is formed besides cholesterol in the mevalonate pathway. The continuous production of small amounts of geranylgeraniol and consequently, a continuous production of cholesterol, in a subgroup of neurons is required for spatial, assocative and motor learning. Interesting is the notification that the decrease in the cholesterol synthesis rate during aging may be associated with an increase in loss of memory functions [49].

In contrast with the expectations lovastatin appeared to induce the deposition of amyloid in brain of an AD-mouse-model, and George *et al* found that diet-induced hypercholesterolemia reduced brain levels of amyloid in aged mice [50].

The beneficial effects of statins on the progression of AD are therefore, most likely not the result of their cholesterol-lowering effect, but may be ascribed to their anti-inflammatory properties or their modulating effects on the vessel wall.

Moreover, LXR-agonists may be promising tools in the treatment of AD. Activation of the LXR-pathway via synthetic agonists was found to reduce the production of amyloid in cultured neurons [51]. It was suggested that this resulted from an up-regulated expression of ABCA1. If this needs to be accompanied by an enhanced neuronal cholesterol efflux remains controversial [51-53]. Also *in vivo* in AD-mice LXR-activation was found to reduce amyloid levels in the brain and in line its deposition [54]. Different molecular mechanisms may underly these observations. As mentioned before, LXR-agonists may exert their effects directly via an effect on neuronal cholesterol metabolism, which may result in a reduced production of amyloid. LXR-activation may also up-regulate the secretion of ApoE-associated lipoproteins from astrocytes which may bind amyloid-beta in the interstitial fluid and thereby prevent its deposition. Another possibility is that LXR-activation results in an enhanced secretion of amyloid-beta from the brain into the circulation via an enhancing effect on the cholesterol-turnover in the brain (unpublished results). It is thought that amyloid-beta is secreted from the brain together with cholesterol [55].

The addition of supplements to the diet could be an alternative strategy to modulate brain cholesterol metabolism, and thereby the development and/or the progression of AD. This may be achieved for example via the addition of specific plant sterols or fatty acids that have been found to affect the LXR-pathway [47,56].

Our present research focusses on the question if modulation of the LXR-pathway can lead to enhanced learning and memory functions and on the prevention, retardation and/or even restoration of neurodegenerative processes in models for AD.

References

[1]   I. Bjorkhem, L. Starck, U. Andersson *et al.* Oxysterols in the circulation of patients with the Smith-Lemli-Opitz syndrome: abnormal levels of 24S- and 27-hydroxycholesterol. *J. Lipid Res.* **42** (2001) 366-371.

[2]   V. Wiegand, T.Y. Chang, J.F. Strauss *et al.* Transport of plasma membrane-derived cholesterol and the function of Niemann-Pick C1 Protein. *FASEB J.* **17** (2003) 782-784.

[3]   M.H. Moghadasian, G. Salen, J.J. Frohlich *et al.* Cerebrotendinous xanthomatosis: a rare disease with diverse manifestations. *Arch. Neurol.* **59** (2002) 527-529.

[4]   J. Marx. Alzheimer's disease. Bad for the heart, bad for the mind? *Science* **294** (2001) 508-509.

[5]   L. Puglielli, B.C. Ellis, L.A. Ingano *et al.* Role of acyl-coenzyme a: cholesterol acyltransferase activity in the processing of the amyloid precursor protein. *J. Mol. Neurosci.* **24** (2004) 93-96.

[6]   J. Edmond, R.A. Korsak, J.W. Morrow *et al.* Dietary cholesterol and the origin of cholesterol in the brain of developing rats. *J. Nutr.* **121** (1991) 1323-1330.

[7]   D. Lutjohann, O. Breuer, G. Ahlborg *et al.* Cholesterol homeostasis in human brain: evidence for an age-dependent flux of 24S-hydroxycholesterol from the brain into the circulation. *Proc. Natl. Acad. Sci. U.S.A.* **93** (1996) 9799-9804.

[8]   I. Bjorkhem, D. Lutjohann, O. Breuer *et al.* Importance of a novel oxidative mechanism for elimination of brain cholesterol. Turnover of cholesterol and 24(S)-hydroxycholesterol in rat brain as measured with 18O2 techniques in vivo and in vitro. *J. Biol. Chem.* **272** (1997) 30178-30184.

[9]   C. Xie, E.G. Lund, S.D. Turley *et al.* Quantitation of two pathways for cholesterol excretion from the brain in normal mice and mice with neurodegeneration. *J. Lipid Res.* **44** (2003) 1780-1789.

[10]   S. Lemaire-Ewing, C. Prunet, T. Montagne *et al.* Comparison of the cytotoxic, pro-oxidant and pro-inflammatory characteristics of different oxysterols. *Cell Biol. Toxicol.* **21** (2005) 97-114.

[11]   C. Travert, S. Carreau, D. Le Goff *et al.* Induction of apoptosis by 25-hydroxycholesterol in adult rat Leydig cells: protective effect of 17beta-estradiol. *Reprod. Toxicol.* **22** (2006) 564-570.

[12]   E.H. Corder, A.M. Saunders, W.J. Strittmatter *et al.* Gene dose of apolipoprotein E type 4 allele and the risk of Alzheimer's disease in late onset families. *Science* **261** (1993) 921-923.

[13]   J. Poirier, J. Davignon, D. Bouthillier *et al.* Apolipoprotein E polymorphism and Alzheimer's disease. *Lancet* **342** (1993) 697-699.

[14]   R.W. Mahley. Apolipoprotein E: cholesterol transport protein with expanding role in cell biology. *Science* **240** (1988) 622-630.

[15]   J. Poirier, A. Baccichet, D. Dea *et al.* Cholesterol synthesis and lipoprotein reuptake during synaptic remodelling in hippocampus in adult rats. *Neuroscience* **55** (1993) 81-90.

[16]   M. Mulder, A. Blokland, D.J. van den Berg *et al.* Apolipoprotein E protects against neuropathology induced by a high-fat diet and maintains the integrity of the blood-brain barrier during aging. *Lab. Invest.* **81** (2001) 953-960.

[17]   B. Wolozin. Cholesterol and the biology of Alzheimer's disease. *Neuron* **41** (2004) 7-10.

[18]   G.P. Eckert, C. Kirsch, W.E. Mueller *et al.* Differential effects of lovastatin treatment on brain cholesterol levels in normal and apoE-deficient mice. *Neuroreport* **12** (2001) 883-887.

[19]   W.B. Grant, A. Campbell, R.F. Itzhaki *et al.* The significance of environmental factors in the etiology of Alzheimer's disease. *J. Alzheimers Dis.* **4** (2002) 179-189.

[20]   D.L. Sparks. Coronary artery disease, hypertension, ApoE, and cholesterol: a link to Alzheimer's disease? *Ann. N.Y. Acad. Sci.* **826** (1997) 128-146.

[21]   J.A. Levin-Allerhand, C.E. Lominska, J.D. Smith. Increased amyloid-levels in APPSWE transgenic mice treated chronically with a physiological high-fat high-cholesterol diet. *J. Nutr. Health Aging* **6** (2002) 315-319.

[22]   M. Oksman, H. Iivonen, E. Hogyes *et al.* Impact of different saturated fatty acid, polyunsaturated fatty acid and cholesterol containing diets on beta-amyloid accumulation in APP/PS1 transgenic mice. *Neurobiol. Dis.* **23** (2006) 563-572.

[23]   T. Mori, D. Paris, T. Town *et al.* Cholesterol accumulates in senile plaques of Alzheimer disease patients and in transgenic APP(SW) mice. *J. Neuropathol. Exp. Neurol.* **60** (2001) 778-785.

[24]   M. Mulder, R. Ravid, D.F. Swaab *et al.* Reduced levels of cholesterol, phospholipids, and fatty acids in cerebrospinal fluid of Alzheimer disease patients are not related to apolipoprotein E4. *Alzheimer Dis. Assoc. Disord.* **12** (1998) 198-203.

[25]   L. Bretillon, D. Lutjohann, L. Stahle *et al.* Plasma levels of 24S-hydroxycholesterol reflect the balance between cerebral production and hepatic metabolism and are inversely related to body surface. *J. Lipid Res.* **41** (2000) 840-845.

[26]   A. Papassotiropoulos, D. Lutjohann, M. Bagli *et al.* 24S-hydroxycholesterol in cerebrospinal fluid is elevated in early stages of dementia. *J. Psychiatr. Res.* **36** (2002) 27-32.

[27]   P. Schonknecht, D. Lutjohann, J. Pantel *et al.* Cerebrospinal fluid 24S-hydroxycholesterol is increased in patients with Alzheimer's disease compared to healthy controls. *Neurosci. Lett.* **324** (2002) 83-85.

[28]   M. Heverin, N. Bogdanovic, D. Lutjohann *et al.* Changes in the levels of cerebral and extracerebral sterols in the brain of patients with Alzheimer's disease. *J. Lipid Res.* **45** (2004) 186-193.

[29]   H. Kolsch, D. Lutjohann, M. Ludwig *et al.* Polymorphism in the cholesterol 24S-hydroxylase gene is associated with Alzheimer's disease. *Mol. Psychiatry* **7** (2002) 899-902.

[30]   E.J. Murphy, H.M. Huang, R.F. Cowburn *et al.* Phospholipid mass is increased in fibroblasts bearing the Swedish amyloid precursor mutation. *Brain Res. Bull.* **69** (2006) 79-85.

[31]   M. Simons, P. Keller, B. De Strooper *et al.* Cholesterol depletion inhibits the generation of beta-amyloid in hippocampal neurons. *Proc. Natl. Acad. Sci. U.S.A.* **95** (1998) 6460-6464.

[32]   E.R. Frears, D.J. Stephens, C.E. Walters *et al.* The role of cholesterol in the biosynthesis of beta-amyloid. *Neuroreport* **10** (1999) 1699-1705.

[33]   L. Puglielli, G. Konopka, E. Pack-Chung *et al.* Acyl-coenzyme A: cholesterol acyltransferase modulates the generation of the amyloid beta-peptide. *Nat. Cell Biol.* **3** (2001) 905-912.

[34]   T. Hartmann. Role of amyloid precursor protein, amyloid-beta and gamma-secretase in cholesterol maintenance. *Neurodegener. Dis.* **3** (2006) 305-311.

[35]   P.J. Jansen, D. Lutjohann, K. Abildayeva *et al.* Dietary plant sterols accumulate in the brain. *Biochim. Biophys. Acta* **1761** (2006) 445-453.

[36]   R.E. Pitas, J.K. Boyles, S.H. Lee *et al.* Lipoproteins and their receptors in the central nervous system. Characterization of the lipoproteins in cerebrospinal fluid and identification of apolipoprotein B,E(LDL) receptors in the brain. *J. Biol. Chem.* **262** (1987) 14352-14360.

[37]   J.S. Gong, M. Kobayashi, H. Hayashi *et al.* Apolipoprotein E (ApoE) isoform-dependent lipid release from astrocytes prepared from human ApoE3 and ApoE4 knock-in mice. *J. Biol. Chem.* **277** (2002) 29919-29926.

[38]   H. Hayashi, R.B. Campenot, D.E. Vance *et al.* Glial lipoproteins stimulate axon growth of central nervous system neurons in compartmented cultures. *J. Biol. Chem.* **279** (2004) 14009-14015.

[39]   E.G. Lund, C. Xie, T. Kotti *et al.* Knockout of the cholesterol 24-hydroxylase gene in mice reveals a brain-specific mechanism of cholesterol turnover. *J. Biol. Chem.* **278** (2003) 22980-22988.

[40]   S.B. Joseph, A. Castrillo, B.A. Laffitte *et al.* Reciprocal regulation of inflammation and lipid metabolism by liver X receptors. *Nat. Med.* **9** (2003) 213-219.

[41]   S.B. Joseph and P. Tontonoz. LXRs: new therapeutic targets in atherosclerosis? *Curr. Opin. Pharmacol.* **3** (2003) 192-197.

[42]   K.D. Whitney, M.A. Watson, J.L. Collins *et al.* Regulation of cholesterol homeostasis by the liver X receptors in the central nervous system. *Mol. Endocrinol.* **16** (2002) 1378-1385.

[43]   L. Wang, G.U. Schuster, K. Hultenby *et al.* Liver X receptors in the central nervous system: from lipid homeostasis to neuronal degeneration. *Proc. Natl. Acad. Sci. U.S.A.* **99** (2002) 13878-13883.

[44]   K. Abildayeva, P.J. Jansen, V. Hirsch-Reinshagen *et al.* 24(S)-hydroxycholesterol participates in a liver X receptor-controlled pathway in astrocytes that regulates apolipoprotein E-mediated cholesterol efflux. *J. Biol. Chem.* **281** (2006) 12799-12808.

[45]   K.M. Thelen, K.M. Rentsch, U. Gutteck *et al.* Brain cholesterol synthesis in mice is affected by high dose of simvastatin but not of pravastatin. *J. Pharmacol. Exp. Ther.* **316** (2006) 1146-1152.

[46]   L. Li, D. Cao, H. Kim *et al.* Simvastatin enhances learning and memory independent of amyloid load in mice. *Ann. Neurol.* **60** (2006) 729-739.

[47]   L.R. Wagstaff, M.W. Mitton, B.M. Arvik *et al.* Statin-associated memory loss: analysis of 60 case reports and review of the literature. *Pharmacotherapy* **23** (2003) 871-880.

[48]   T.J. Kotti, D.M. Ramirez, B.E. Pfeiffer *et al.* Brain cholesterol turnover required for geranylgeraniol production and learning in mice. *Proc. Natl. Acad. Sci. U.S.A.* **103** (2006) 3869-3874.

[49]   K.M. Thelen, P. Falkai, T.A. Bayer *et al.* Cholesterol synthesis rate in human hippocampus declines with aging. *Neurosci. Lett.* **403** (2006) 15-19.

[50]   A.J. George, R.M. Holsinger, C.A. McLean *et al.* APP intracellular domain is increased and soluble Abeta is reduced with diet-induced hypercholesterolemia in a transgenic mouse model of Alzheimer disease. *Neurobiol. Dis.* **16** (2004) 124-132.

[51]   Y. Sun, J. Yao, T.W. Kim *et al.* Expression of liver X receptor target genes decreases cellular amyloid beta peptide secretion. *J. Biol. Chem.* **278** (2003) 27688-27694.

[52]   G.W. Rebeck. Cholesterol efflux as a critical component of Alzheimer's disease pathogenesis. *J. Mol. Neurosci.* **23** (2004) 219-224.

[53]   M.P. Burns, L. Vardanian, A. Pajoohesh-Ganji *et al.* The effects of ABCA1 on cholesterol efflux and Abeta levels in vitro and in vivo. *J. Neurochem.* **98** (2006) 792-800.

[54]   R.P. Koldamova, I.M. Lefterov, M. Staufenbiel *et al.* The liver X receptor ligand T0901317 decreases amyloid beta production in vitro and in a mouse model of Alzheimer's disease. *J. Biol. Chem.* **280** (2005) 4079-4088.

[55]   M. Mulder and D. Terwel. Possible link between lipid metabolism and cerebral amyloid angiopathy in Alzheimer's disease: A role for high-density lipoproteins? *Haemostasis* **28** (1998) 174-194.

[56]   C. Yang, L. Yu, W. Li *et al.* Disruption of cholesterol homeostasis by plant sterols. *J. Clin. Invest.* **114** (2004) 813-822.

Nuclear Receptors as Molecular Targets for Cardiometabolic and Central Nervous System Diseases
J.L. Junien and B. Staels (Eds.)
IOS Press, 2008

93

PPARγ-Mediated Effects in CNS Disorders

Stephan A. Paxian, Lars Tatenhorst, Michael T. Heneka
Department of Neurology, Molecular Neurology Unit, University of Münster, Albert Schweitzer-Strasse 33, 48149 Münster, Germany

Abstract. The biology and role of peroxisome proliferator-activated receptors (PPARs) for physiological and pathophysiological processes has been primarily studied in peripherial organs and tissues. Little is known about the physiological role of PPARs for brain development, maintainance and function. Lessions from transgenic mouse models, however, provide evidence that PPARs may play pivotal roles for CNS development and performance. Thus, knock-out of the PPARβ/δ isoform results in disconnection of the two brain hemispheres and the expression pattern of PPARγ in late fetal development points to an important role for CNS development.

Recently it became clear, that PPARs play an important role for the pathogenesis of various disorders of the CNS. The finding that activation of PPARs, and in particular of the PPARγ isoform, suppresses inflammation in peripherial macrophages and in models of human autoimmune disease, instigated the experimental evaluation of these salutary actions for several CNS disorders that harbor an inflammatory component. Activation of all PPAR isoforms, but especially of PPARγ, has been found to be protective in murine *in vitro* and *in vivo* models of Multiple Sclerosis. The verification of these findings in human cells prompted the initiation of clinical studies evaluating PPARγ activation in Multiple Sclerosis patients. Likewise, Alzheimer's disease (AD) has a prominent inflammatory component that arises in response to neurodegeneration and in particular to extracellular deposition of β-amyloid peptides. The fact that non-steroidal anti-inflammatory drugs (NSAIDs) delay the onset and reduce the risk to develop AD, while they also bind to and activate PPARγ, led to the hypothesis that one dimension of NSAID protection in AD may be mediated by PPARγ. Several lines of evidence from *in vitro* and *in vivo* studies have supported this hypothesis, using AD-related transgenic cellular and animal models. Principally, anti-amyloidogenic, anti-inflammatory and insulin-sensitizing effects may account for the observed effects. A number of clinical trials have been communicated with promising results and further trials are in preparation, which aim to delineate the exact mechanism of interaction. Animal models of other neurodegenerative disease such as Parkinson's and Amyotrophic Lateral Sclerosis, both associated with a considerable degree of CNS inflammation, have been studied with a positive outcome. Yet, it is not clear whether reduction of inflammation or other, to date unknown mechanisms, account for the observed neuroprotection.

Keywords. Alzheimer's disease, Multiple Sclerosis, Parkinson's disease, Amyotrophic Lateral Sclerosis, ischemic stroke

Introduction

Physiological Function of PPARs in the Brain

The peroxisome proliferator-activated receptors (PPARs) are ligand-inducible transcription factors which belong to the superfamily of phylogenetically related proteins termed nuclear hormone receptors (NHR). As with other members of the NHR superfamily, comprising steroid, thyroid and retinoid receptors, it is thought that the ability of PPARs to bind to a ligand was acquired during metazoan evolution since these proteins are present in all metazoan phyla. Three different PPAR isotypes (PPARα, PPARβ, also called δ, and PPARγ) have been identified in various species. In rodents, PPARα, PPARβ and PPARγ show unique spatio-temporal tissue-dependent patterns of expression during fetal development in a broad range of cell-types having ectodermal, mesodermal or endodermal embryonic origins. PPARs are involved in several aspects of tissue differentiation and rodent development, such as the differentiation of the adipose tissue, brain, placenta and skin (reviewed in [1]). Therefore, it appears that PPARα, β and γ developed from a common PPAR with broad ligand-binding specificity, itself derived from the ancestral orphan receptor (reviewed in [2]).

PPARs regulate gene expression through multiple mechanisms and function as obligate heterodimers with Retinoid X Receptors (RXRs). Like the other members of the superfamily, PPARs are composed of four domains. The DNA-binding domain is highly conserved and its zinc finger domain is a common attribute of all members of the NHR superfamily. The DNA-binding domain is linked to the C-terminal ligand-binding domain by the hinge region. The E/F domain is responsible for the dimerization of PPARs with RXRs and the ligand-dependent transactivation function of the receptor, whereas the N-terminal domain is involved in the ligand-independent regulation of the receptor activity (reviewed in [3]).

PPARs bind to conserved DNA sequences termed peroxisome proliferator response elements (PPREs) present in the promoter of target genes. In the absence of ligands, these heterodimers are physically associated with co-repressor complexes which block gene transcription [1]. In the presence of a ligand, these heterodimers associate with co-activator complexes, thereby activating gene transcription. PPARs are also competent in regulating gene expression independent of binding to PPREs. PPARγ agonists are believed to suppress immune responses principally through transrepression. Some agonists have been shown to inhibit transcription factors including AP-1, STAT-1 and nuclear factor κB (NFκB) from activating gene expression in a dose-dependent manner [4,5].

PPARs were initially reported to be induced by peroxisome proliferators, a group of substances able to activate peroxisome proliferation. For now, various endogenous and exogenous PPAR ligands were identified, including fatty acids, eicosanoids, synthetic hypolipidemic and anti-diabetic agents (reviewed in [3]). Most of the PPAR target genes are involved in various steps of lipid metabolism and energy homeostasis, which highlights the importance of these receptors in vertebrate physiology (reviewed in [6]). The best characterized functions of PPARs are the role of PPARα in fatty acid catabolism in the liver, and the opposite but complementary role of PPARγ in adipogenesis and fatty acid metabolism and lipid storage. However, in addition to these functions, which are key regulators in the maintenance of the energy balance in adult animals, PPARs were demonstrated to be implicated in distinct aspects of rodent development (reviewed in [7]).

Binding of PPARs to their specific ligands leads to conformational changes which allow co-repressor release and co-activator recruitment. Even though all PPARs can be attributed to a common ancestral nuclear receptor, each PPAR isotype has its own properties with regard to ligand binding. Synthetic thiazolidinediones (TZDs), which are commonly prescribed for the treatment of type-2 diabetes, are selective PPARγ ligands. Naturally occurring PPARγ ligands include eicosanoids and the cyclopentenone prostaglandin 15d-PGJ$_2$. The best charcterized PPARγ agonists are the TZDs including troglitazone (Rezulin), pioglitazone (Actos) and rosiglitazone (Avandia) which are Food and Drug Association (FDA) approved for treatment of type-2 diabetes. There is a number of non-TZD based PPARγ agonists, such as GW78456, that have been developed. PPARα ligands include fibrates that are commonly used for the treatment of hypertriglyceridemia and the synthetic agonists WY14,643 and GW7647. PPARβ/δ agonists include the prostacyclin PGI$_2$, and synthetic agents including GW0742, GW501516, and GW7842. All three PPAR isotypes can be activated by polyunsaturated fatty acids with different affinities and efficiencies [8].

PPARα and γ transcripts appear late during fetal development of rat and mouse (day 13.5 of gestation), with a pattern of expression similar to their adult distribution. PPARα is found in the liver, the kidney, the intestine, the heart, the skeletal muscle, the adrenal gland and the pancreas. PPARγ expression is restricted to the brown adipose tissue (day 18.5 of gestation), and to the CNS (day 13.5 to 15.5 of gestation). Compared to the two other isotypes, PPARβ/δ is expressed ubiquitously and earlier during fetal development [9]. In rodent adult organs, the distribution of PPARα is similar to its fetal pattern of expression. In summary, PPARα is expressed in cells with high catabolic rates of fatty acids and peroxisomal metabolism, such as in hepatocytes and cardiomyocytes. PPARγ remains restricted to the brown and white adipose tissue, and is expressed at lower levels in the intestinal mucosa, the retina, the skeletal muscle and lymphoid organs. Similar to its fetal distribution, the PPARβ/δ transcript is present in all organs tested, and is often more abundant than the PPARα and γ transcripts [10].

The expression of the three PPAR isotypes peaks in the rat CNS between day 13.5 and 18.5 of gestation. Whereas PPARβ/δ remains highly expressed in this tissue, the expression of PPARα and γ decreases postnatally in this organ [11].

Little is known about the expression of the PPARs during human development [12-14]. These data show that human PPARα is expressed in the adult liver, heart, kidney, large intestine and skeletal muscle. PPARβ/δ mRNA is present ubiquitously, with a higher expression in the digestive tract and the placenta. PPARγ is abundantly expressed in the white adipose tissue, and is present at lower levels in the skeletal muscle, the heart and the liver. Surprisingly, and in contrast to rodents, human PPARγ seems to be absent from lymphoid tissues, even though PPARγ has been shown to be present in macrophages in human atheroma.

Relatively high levels of PPARγ are found in white and brown adipose tissue, and the importance of PPARγ in adipogenesis has been extensively studied and well documented (reviewed in [15]). Due to the lethality of the PPARγ$^{-/-}$ embryos, alternative mouse models were constructed to study the role of PPARγ *in vivo*. In one of these models, a PPARγ null mouse surviving to term was obtained after selective rescue of the placental defect. In these animals, brown and white adipose tissue was absent, whereas the heterozygous mice developed both types of adipose tissues. The phenotype of PPARβ/δ null mice supports the hypothesis, that PPARβ/δ is a key player in adipocyte differentiation upon stimulation by long-chain fatty acids, since these mice appeared to have reduced fat stores [16].

All three PPAR isotypes are co-expressed in the nervous system during late rat embryogenesis, and PPARβ/δ is the prevalent isotype. During postnatal maturation and in adult animals, only PPARβ/δ remains expressed at significant levels in this tissue. In retina, all three receptors are expressed [11,17,18]. Even though this pattern of expression, which is isotype-specific and regulated during development, suggests that the PPARs may play a role during the formation of the CNS, their function in this tissue is still poorly understood. Both *in vitro* and *in vivo* observations show that PPARβ/δ is the prevalent isoform in the brain, and is found in all cell-types, whereas PPARα is expressed at very low levels predominantly in astrocytes [19]. Acyl-CoA synthetase 2, which is crucial in fatty acid utilization, is regulated by PPARβ/δ at the transcriptional level, providing a facile measure of PPARβ/δ action. This observation strongly suggests that PPARβ/δ participates in the regulation of lipid metabolism in the brain. This hypothesis is further supported by the observation that PPARβ/δ null mice exhibit an altered myelination of the corpus callosum. Such a defect was not observed in other regions of the CNS, and the expression of mRNA encoding proteins involved in the myelination process remained unchanged in the brain [20].

All PPARs, including PPARγ, have been described in the adult and developing brain as well as in the spinal cord. Furthermore, it has been suggested that PPAR activation in neurons may directly influence neuron cell viability and differentiation [21-25]. While PPARβ/δ has been found in neurons of numerous brain areas, PPARα and γ have been localized to more restricted brain areas [26,27]. The localization of PPARs has also been investigated in purified cultures of neural cells. PPARβ/δ is expressed in immature oligodendrocytes, where its activation promotes differentiation, myelin maturation and turnover [28,29]. The γ isotype is the dominant isoform in microglia. Astrocytes possess all three PPAR isotypes, although to different degrees depending on the brain area and animal age [18,30]. The role of PPARs in the CNS is mainly been related to lipid metabolism, however, these receptors have been implicated in neural cell differentiation and death as well as in inflammation and neurodegeneration. The expression of PPARγ in the brain has been extensively studied in relation to inflammation and neurodegeneration [22]. PPARα has been suggested to be involved in the acetylcholine metabolism [31] and to be related to excitatory amino-acid neurotransmission and oxidative stress defense [26].

Role of PPARs in Neuro-immunological Disease

Multiple Sclerosis and Experimental Allergic Encephalitis

Multiple Sclerosis (MS) is a chronic autoimmune disorder of the CNS that begins most commonly in young adults and is characterized pathologically by multiple areas of white matter inflammation, demyelination and glial scarring (sclerosis). It is well accepted that pro-inflammatory cytokines play a key role in the pathogenesis of MS and experimental autoimmune encephalitis (EAE), an established animal model of MS [32]. Several cytokines including tumor necrosis factor α (TNFα), interferon γ (IFNγ), and interleukin 6 (IL-6) are regularly found in MS brain lesions and in spinal cord infiltrates of EAE mice. The fact that PPARγ agonists exert profound and long-lasting anti-inflammatory effects in peripherial immune cells [33-35] and in models of autoimmune disorders including inflammatory bowel disease [36], psoriasis [37] and adjuvant-induced arthritis [38], instigated the experimental use of these drugs in *in vitro* and *in vivo* models of MS. Moreover it has been demonstrated that expression of PPARγ increases in microglia and astrocytes during EAE, supporting a role of this receptor in modulating inflammatory responses in MS [39].

PPARγ in EAE

Using the synthetic PPARγ ligand troglitazone, Niino *et al* first demonstrated in the myelin oligodendrocyte glycoprotein peptide 35-55 (MOG$_{35-55}$)-induced EAE model that activation of PPARγ limits the development of clinical symptoms and infiltration of brain parenchyma by peripheral leukocytes [40]. While this study failed to detect any significant differences in antigen specific T-cell proliferation between troglitazone-treated and untreated mice *in vitro*, it showed that troglitazone treatment significantly decreased TNFα mRNA transcription. Interestingly, Niino *et al* showed that treatment with troglitazone increased the mRNA levels of PPARγ₁ [40]. The potential therapeutic implication of this finding was further supported by a study of Diab *et al* showing that the endogenous PPARγ ligand 15d-PGJ₂ inhibited T-cell proliferation and suppressed IFNγ, IL-10 and IL-4 generation by activated lymphocytes [39]. However, while 15d-PGJ₂ was initially thought to act as a PPARγ agonist, it is now apparent that the dominant action of 15d-PGJ₂ is to directly inhibit IKK, a key enzyme for the initiation of NFκB signalling as well as modification of IκB [5]. It is presently not clear whether 15d-PGJ₂-mediated protection is due to PPARγ activation or IKK inhibition. Feinstein and colleagues were then the first to show that oral pioglitzone treatment of MOG₃₅₋₅₅ immunized mice not only reduced brain inflammation and leukocyte infiltration, but protected from axonal demyelination [41]. While pioglitazone protected in both, monophasic and remittent EAE models in this study, the important finding was that the drug, even when given at the peak of the clinical disease, led to a rapid improvement of symptoms [41]. Interestingly, rosiglitazone did not show a similar protection from clinical EAE symptoms as pioglitazone or GW7845 within the first two weeks of MOG₃₅₋₅₅-induced EAE, a phenomenon that may be explained by the limited blood-brain barrier penetration of this substance. As shown for 15d-PGJ₂, pioglitazone suppressed the IFNγ secretion of splenic T-cells stimulated by MOG₃₅₋₅₅ *in vitro* [41].

In EAE and MS, inflammatory activation of resident endothelial and glial cells as well as infiltrating leukocytes contribute to demyelination and destruction. The entry of peripherial cells into the CNS is stimulated and modulated by the release of chemotactic cytokines (chemokines) (for review see [42]). PPARγ agonists have been shown to reduce the expression of the monocytic chemoattractant MCP1 [43], IP10 (CXCL3), MIG and I-TAC [44]. Supporting the hypothesis that a suppressed generation of chemotactic molecules contributes to the reduced infiltration observed in response to treatment with synthetic PPARγ ligands troglitazone and pioglitazone, a decrease in the mRNA levels for MIP1α and RANTES, both key chemokines in the MOG₃₅₋₅₅-induced EAE model, has been observed [41]. Most of these studies were either performed with synthetic PPARγ agonists or 15d-PGJ₂, this latter compound can act principally by PPARγ-independent mechanisms [45]. However, Bright and colleagues reported that PPARγ-deficient heterozygous (PPARγ(+/-)) mice developed an exacerbated phenotype in the EAE model [46], supporting the hypothesis that the observed effects are indeed due to PPARγ activation. In particular the PPARγ(+/-) mice revealed an increased and prolonged phase of clinical symptoms, more inflammation and demyelination of spinal cord sections and an increase in T-cell proliferation and Th1 response upon MOG peptide stimulation when compared to PPARγ wild-type littermate controls. In a very recent report, Raikwar and colleagues found that PPARγ antagonists, bisphenol A diglycidyl ether and 2-chloro-5-nitro-N-(4 pyridyl)benzamide reversed the suppression of EAE by the PPARγ agonists ciglitazone [47], providing further evidence for PPARγ-dependent TZD effects in murine EAE.

Human Multiple Sclerosis

Since cytokine expression in peripheral blood mononuclear cells (PBMCs) from MS patients correlates well with disease activity and precedes the onset of clinical symptoms up to 4 weeks [48], experimental modulation of PBMC proliferation and inflammatory reaction upon immunostimulation is a useful tool to investigate possible treatment options for this disorder. Schmidt and colleagues compared the immunomodulatory effects of pioglitazone and ciglitazone and the non-thiazolidinedione PPARγ agonist GW347845 on human T-leukemia cells (Jurkat cells) and phytohemaglutinin (PHA)-stimulated PBMCs derived from 21 MS patients and 12 healthy donors [49]. In this study all drugs suppressed PHA-induced T-cell proliferation by 40-50% and secretion of IFNγ and TNFα by 30-50%. However, when PBMCs were pre-incubated with PPARγ agonists for 48 hours, inhibition of proliferation and cytokine secretion were completely abolished, indicating a sensitizing effect of PPARγ activation. The anti-proliferative effects of pioglitazone and GW347845 were accompanied by a decrease of cell viability. Electron microscopy and Western blot analysis revealed DNA condensation and down-regulation of bcl-2 suggesting the induction of apoptosis in activated T-lymphocytes [49].

As a striking finging, anti-inflammatory effects of pioglitazone treatment were significantly reduced in MS patients when compared to healthy controls. Surprisingly PBMCs from MS patients exhibited a strong reduction in PPARγ expression [50]. Furthermore, inflammatory stimulation of PBMCs from healthy controls resulted in loss of PPARγ, a phenomenon that was previously observed in adipocytes and bone marrow stromal cells [51-53]. Co-incubation with pioglitazone did not prevent the inflammation-induced loss of PPARγ, while pre-incubation with the drug stabilized PPARγ levels. Importantly, long-term oral pioglitazone treatment prevented the PHA-induced loss of PPARγ expression in PBMCs from diabetic patients, demonstrating that the concentrations of pioglitazone achieved by a standard oral treatment in humans are sufficient to protect from inflammation-induced loss of PPARγ. Reporter gene assays revealed increased PPARγ$_1$ promoter activity after pioglitazone pre-incubation. These results suggest that after inflammatory stimulation PPARγ$_1$ promoter activity is suppressed resulting in decreased PPARγ expression levels. Significantly, this inflammation-induced decrease in PPARγ expression can be prevented either by pre-incubation with pioglitazone *in vitro* or by oral treatment with pioglitazone as demonstrated in PBMCs derived from diabetic patients. Differences in PPARγ expression and promoter activity were accompanied by changes in PPARγ DNA-binding activity, as pre-incubation with pioglitazone increased DNA-binding of PPARγ. Additionally, pre-incubation decreased NFκB DNA-binding activity to control levels, while the levels of the inhibitory protein, IκBα, were increased. In MS patients, pioglitazone-induced increase in PPARγ DNA-binding activity and corresponding decrease in NFκB DNA-binding activity was only observed in the absence of an acute MS relapse. These results suggest that the sensitizing effect observed in the pre-incubation experiments is mediated by prevention of inflammation-induced suppression of PPARγ expression with consecutive increase in PPARγ DNA-binding activity.

The aforementioned *in vitro* and *in vivo* experiments suggest that PPAR activation may be used as a new therapeutic avenue in the treatment of MS. Treatment of a single patient with pioglitazone has been reported as an index case [54]. In this report, oral pioglitazone treatment increased the body weight along with an improved motor strength and coordination. There were no adverse events and the clinical benefits were persistent over the entire observation period of three years in this patient.

Role of PPARs in Neurodegenerative Disorders

Alzheimer's Disease

Alzheimer's disease (AD) is the most common cause of dementia. The number of individuals with the disease is dramatically increasing throughout the developed world. The large number of affected individuals and the increasing prevalence of the disease present a substantial challenge to health care systems and do so in the face of substantial economic costs. The drugs that are now in use to treat the disease are principally targeted at symptomatic improvement of the patients. These agents typically have modest therapeutic efficacy over rather short periods. Moreover, only a subset of patients responds positively to this therapy. Thus, the development of new therapeutic approaches to the disease is of critical importance.

PPARγ agonists have been advanced as a new therapeutic and disease process altering approach to AD. Several different mechanisms have been postulated to account for the actions of PPARγ agonists in AD. The initial studies exploring the actions of PPARγ in AD were based on the ability of non-steroidal anti-inflammatory drugs to activate this receptor. There are a number of compelling epidemiological studies that demonstrate the NSAID treatment reduces AD risk by as much as 80% and it was suggested that these effects might arise from the ability of these drugs to stimulate PPARγ activation and to inhibit inflammatory responses in the AD brain [55-58]. AD has a significant inflammatory component, which has been associated with amyloidosis and neuronal loss [59] and proposed as a future therapeutic target [60]. Amyloid plaques within the brain are populated by abundant, activated microglia and astrocytes. In addition, neuronal expression of inflammatory enzyme systems including iNOS has been described in AD [61-63]. The experimental expression of iNOS in neurons resulted in time-dependent neuronal cell death which was prevented by activation of PPARγ *in vitro* and *in vivo* [22,64]. PPARγ activation in microglial cells suppressed inflammatory cytokine expression, iNOS expression and NO production and inhibition of COX2 and subsequent generation of immunostimulated prostanoid synthesis [65].

These latter effects are a result of the ability of PPARγ to suppress the promoters of pro-inflammatory genes through antagonism of the actions of the transcription factors NFκB, AP-1 and STAT [66]. PPARγ agonists have been demonstrated suppress the Aβ-mediated activation of microglia *in vitro* and prevent cortical or hippocampal neuronal cell death [65,67,68]. In a rat model of cortical Aβ injection, co-injection of ciglitazone and ibuprofen or oral administration of pioglitazone potently suppressed acute Aβ-evoked microglial cytokine generation. Interestingly, all PPARγ agonists used in this study increased the levels of IκBα and IκBβ and finally reduced the nuclear translocation of NFκB [69].

The effects of the PPARγ agonists have been investigated in animal models of AD that over-express human APP. These initial studies employed the PPARγ agonist pioglitazone as it is reported to pass the blood-brain barrier (BBB), although its penetrance is limited [70]. The first reported study used the Tg2576 mice one year of age, which were then treated for 6 months with oral pioglitazone. Drug treatment was associated with a small reduction in soluble Aβ levels with no effect on Aβ plaque levels or inflammatory markers [71]. The modest effects of pioglitazone in this study were thought to be due to poor drug penetrance into the brain. A subsequent study by Heneka *et al* found that treatment with a significantly larger dose of pioglitazone in APPV717I transgenic mice at one year of age resulted in a profound reduction of activated microglia and astrocytes and a significantly reduced Aβ plaque burden [72]. The finding that PPARγ agonists elicited a reduction in amyloid pathology in animal models of the disease may be the result of the ability of PPARγ to affect Aβ homeostasis. It has recently been reported that PPARγ agonists inhibit Aβ production that is stimulated by inflammatory cytokines. Sastre *et al* provided evident that this effect was the result of inhibition of beta secretease (BACE1) expression through a PPARγ-dependent suppression of the BACE gene promoter [73,74]. In line with this, Heneka *et al* found that oral pioglitazone treatment of APP transgenic mice reduced BACE1 transcription and expression [72]. A series of independent studies found that PPARγ activation regulated both cellular APP levels and Aβ production by stimulating the ubiquitin-mediated degradation of APP [75]. A recent study has found that

PPARγ is associated with enhanced Aβ clearance [76]. Camacho and colleagues reported that PPARγ activation, in both glia and neurons, led to the rapid and robust uptake of Aβ, leading to its clearance from the medium. The cellular mechanisms that are responsible for this effect are yet unknown [76].

Pedersen and colleagues have demonstrated that rosiglitazone treatment of Tg2576 mice results in improved behavioral performance. They found that treatment with rosiglitazone for 4 months resulted in enhanced spatial working and reference memory [77]. Significantly, drug treatment was associated with a 25% reduction in $A\beta_{1-42}$ levels, however, $A\beta_{1-40}$ levels were unaffected. The reduced $A\beta_{1-42}$ was argued to arise from an increase in the levels of insulin degrading enzyme (IDE) in rosiglitazone-treated transgenic mice. IDE acts to proteolytically degrade amyloid peptides and has been genetically linked to AD [78].

The outcome of two clinical trials of the PPARγ agonist rosiglitazone in AD have recently been reported [79,80]. These studies reported that rosiglitazone therapy improves cognition in a subset of AD patients. Rosiglitazone does not pass the BBB [79,81], and this has been a confound in interpreting the CNS actions resulting from the administration of this drug. These data were interpreted as evidence for a significant role for peripheral insulin sensitivity in cognition. AD risk and memory impairment is associated with hyperinsulinemia, and insulin resistance features which characterize type-2 diabetes [82,83]. Indeed, type-2 diabetes is associated with increased risk of AD [82,84]. These linkages led to the initiation of clinical investigations of insulin-sensitizing TZDs currently in clinical use for the treatment of type-2 diabetes. The results are a pilot clinical trial examining the effects of 6 months of treatment with rosiglitazone on cognition and memory in AD patients [80]. This small study of 30 patients with mild AD or MCI found that rosiglitazone therapy resulted in improved memory and selective attention. A pilot clinical trial of pioglitazone in AD patients has been completed [85]. A large trial of rosiglitazone in AD patients has recently been reported [79]. Risner *et al* examined the effect of rosiglitazone treatment in more than 500 patients with mild to moderate AD. The patients were treated for 6 months with rosiglitazone [79]. Drug treatment resulted in a statistically significant improvement in cognition in those patients that did not possess an ApoE4 allele. Patients with ApoE4 did not respond to the drug and showed no improvement in standard cognitive tests. Risner *et al* suggested that rosiglitazone acts on mitochondria in the brain, increasing their metabolic efficiency and number [79]. This explanation remains unsatisfying as there is no evidence that peripherally delivered rosiglitazone can directly act in the brain. The actions of TZDs on mitochondria are largely PPARγ-independent (see review [86]). This hypothesis is reliant upon penetrance of the drug into the brain and this is problematic as rosiglitazone does not pass the BBB [80,87]. The basis of the differential effects of rosiglitazone in individuals depending on their ApoE genotype is unexplained. The outcome of this clinical trial is, however, consistent with previous findings with respect to the influence of the ApoE4 genotype [88-90].

Parkinson's Disease

Parkinson's disease (PD) is a disabelling age-related, degenerative movement disorder of the CNS that is characterized clinically by tremor, bradykinesia and rigidity and disturbed postural reflexes. The pathological hallmark of idiopathic PD is the loss of dopaminergic neurons in the substantia nigra *pars compacta*. Excitotoxicity, oxidative phosphorylation, the production of reactive oxygen intermediates (ROIs) and apoptosis may significantly contribute to neuronal cell degeneration. Insights into the pathogenesis of PD have been achieved experimentally by using the neurotoxin 1-methyl-4-phenyl-1,2,3,6-tetrahydropyridine (MPTP) in mice. It has been shown that NO acts as an important mediator of MPTP toxicity in dopaminergic neurons [91-93]. Further studies suggested that neuro-inflammatory changes accompanied by microglial and astroglial iNOS expression, may play a pivotal role in Parkinson's disease [94] and MPTP-induced toxicity [95,96]. Since PPARγ activation results in a profound suppression of iNOS in peripheral macrophages [33,35], as well as in models of neuro-inflammation [22,69], MPTP-treated mice were treated with synthetic PPARγ ligands to test the hypothesis that PPARγ-mediated anti-inflammatory effects would exert neuroprotection. Breidert and colleagues found that pioglitazone treatment protected from MPTP-induced dopaminergic cell death in the substantia nigra *pars compacta* [97]. This finding was confirmed by Dehmer and colleagues who demonstrated PPARγ expression in the striatum and the substantia nigra in vehicle- and MPTP-treated mice [98]. In this study, pioglitazone also protected tyrosine hydroxylase-positive substantia nigra neurons from MPTP-induced cell death. However, in both studies, the decrease in striatal dopamine was only partially prevented. Pioglitazone decreased microglial and astrocyte activation and reduced the number of iNOS-positive cells in both the striatum and substantia nigra *pars compacta* [97,98]. In part, iNOS suppression in MPTP-treated mice may have been achieved by reduced NFκB-dependent signal transduction, since pioglitazone treatment induced a striatal increase of IκBα, a direct inhibitor of NFκB nuclear translocation.

Recent evidence suggested that medication with NSAIDs, and in particular ibuprofen, may delay or prevent the development of PD [99,100] through mechanism similar to NSAID protection in AD (see above). Since Ibuprofen passess the BBB and potentially acts as a PPARγ agonist [101] it is possible that PPAR activation contributes to the observed beneficial effect on PD epidemiology. Taken together, these data suggest that treatment with PPARγ agonists may offer a new therapeutic avenue in the treatment of Parkinson's disease.

Amyotrophic Lateral Sclerosis

Amyotrophic Lateral Sclerosis (ALS) represents a fatal neurodegenerative disorder characterized by progressive death of the upper and lower motor neuron. Because increasing evidence suggested that accompanying inflammation may interact with and promote neurodegeneration [102,103], anti-inflammatory treatment strategies are being evaluated in transgenic mouse models of ALS. As for AD, it has been the potent anti-inflammatory action of PPARγ agonists that prompted experiments which tested whether SOD1-G93A transgenic mice, an established mouse model of ALS, benefit from oral treatment with the PPARγ agonist pioglitazone [104,105]. Both studies independently found that oral treatment with the PPARγ agonist pioglitazone extended the survival of SOD1-G93A mice. Pioglitazone treatment delayed the onset of disease and prevented the decrease of body weight in comparison to untreated SOD1-G93A mice. Quantification of motor neurons of the spinal cord revealed neuroprotection by pioglitazone, whereas non-treated SOD1-G93A mice had lost 30%-40% of motor neurons at a comparable time point of the disease [104,105]. This was paralleled by preservation of the median fiber diameter of the quadriceps muscle indicating not only morphological but also functional protection of motor neurons by pioglitazone [105]. This finding was further substantiated by improved motor performance in the Rotarod test [104] and in the grip latency test [105]. Activated microglia were significantly reduced at sites of neurodegeneration in pioglitazone-treated SOD1-G93A mice, as were the protein levels of COX2 and iNOS. Kiaei *et al* also provided evidence that NO-dependent peroxynitrite generation was reduced in response to pioglitazone [104]. Interestingly, mRNA levels of the suppressor of cytokine signalling 1 and 3 genes were increased by pioglitazone, whereas both the mRNA and protein levels of endogenous mouse SOD1 and of transgenic human SOD1 remained unaffected [105].

While the underlying mechanisms may not be fully understood yet, together, both studies suggested that ALS patients may benefit from treatment with this PPARγ agonist. The fact that pioglitazone has been approved for the treatment of type-2 diabetes has prompted a first clinical trial (GERPALS, german pioglitazone study in ALS) which started to enroll patients late 2006.

PPARs in Cerebral Ischemia

Stroke and ischemic damage to the brain is one of the major causes of disability and there are few therapeutic options available for these patients. Ischemic damage arises from impaired blood flow to the brain and elicits the immediate recruitment of neutrophils within a few minutes followed by infiltration of the ischemic tissue by monocytes/macrophages to the site of damage over the next few hours [106]. Ischemia also results in the activation of endogenous microglia in the first hours following the insult. The peripheral leukocytes and microglia mount a robust inflammatory response with the induction of cytokine and chemokine expression as well as elevated expression of adhesion molecules, iNOS, COX2 and other inflammatory mediators which act to exacerbate the tissue damage [107-109]. Importantly, a number of studies have demonstrated that suppression of the inflammatory response ameliorates stroke damage and improves clinical outcomes [110-114]. In line with the above mentioned neurological disorders, the rationale for the use of PPARγ agonists arises principally from the anti-inflammatory actions of these drugs [115].

Experimental Stroke Models

Sundararajan and colleagues first demonstrated that treatment with three different TZD PPARγ agonists, administered intraperitoneally, resulted in reduced infarct volumes and improved sensorimotor function in a rodent middle cerebral artery occlusion (MCAO) [116,117]. The salutary action of the drugs was associated with reduced infiltration of peripheral leukocytes, diminished microglial activation and reduction of iNOS, COX2 and cytokine expression. Similar effects were observed following oral [118] or intracerebrovascular [119] drug administration. The effects of PPARγ agonists have been shown to be due to direct effects on PPARγ [120] and are exhibited by both TZD and non-TZD PPARγ agonists [120]. A number of additional studies have validated these findings [121-124].

The principal focus of studies of PPAR agonists have been on agonists of the PPARγ isoform, however, Deplanque *et al* reported that chronic treatment with the PPARα agonist fenfibrate conferred reduced susceptibility to stroke and reduced infarct size [125]. PPARα agonists were also reported to reduce stroke-related oxidative damage [126]. Recently Arsenijevic and colleagues have explored the role of PPARβ/δ in stroke and found that PPARβ/δ null mice exhibited significantly greater infarct sizes than wild-type animals, suggesting a neuroprotective role for this receptor and that its agonists may be of utility in stroke [127].

Epidemiology and Clinical Evidence

The outcome of a large clinical trial (PROactive) has recently been reported and demonstrated that pioglitazone significantly reduces the combined risk of heart attacks, strokes and death by 16% in high risk patients with type-2 diabetes [128]. A small clinical trial has revealed that diabetic patients receiving pioglitazone or rosiglitazone showed improved functional recovery after stroke compared to patients not receiving TZD therapy

[129]. An NIH sponsored trial is currently testing the ability of pioglitazone to decrease stroke incidence in non-diabetic patients with insulin resistance. A recent report suggests that the Pro12Ala polymorphism of PPARγ$_2$ is associated with a reduced risk for ischemic stroke [130], further supporting the importance of PPARs in cerebral ischemia.

References

[1]   B. Desvergne and W. Wahli. Peroxisome proliferator-activated receptors: nuclear control of metabolism. *Endocr. Rev.* **20** (1999) 649-688.

[2]   H. Escriva, F. Delaunay, V. Laudet. Ligand binding and nuclear receptor evolution. *Bioessays* **22** (2000) 717-727.

[3]   S. Kersten and W. Wahli. Peroxisome proliferator activated receptor agonists. *EXS* **89** (2000) 141-151.

[4]   A. Castrillo, M.J. Diaz-Guerra, S. Hortelano *et al.* Inhibition of IkappaB kinase and IkappaB phosphorylation by 15-deoxy-Delta(12,14)-prostaglandin J(2) in activated murine macrophages. *Mol. Cell. Biol.* **20** (2000) 1692-1698.

[5]   A. Rossi, P. Kapahi, G. Natoli *et al.* Anti-inflammatory cyclopentenone prostaglandins are direct inhibitors of IkappaB kinase. *Nature* **403** (2000) 103-108.

[6]   P. Escher and W. Wahli. Peroxisome proliferator-activated receptors: insight into multiple cellular functions. *Mutat. Res.* **448** (2000) 121-138.

[7]   L. Michalik, B. Desvergne, C. Dreyer *et al.* PPAR expression and function during vertebrate development. *Int. J. Dev. Biol.* **46** (2002) 105-114.

[8]   G. Krey, O. Braissant, F. L'Horset *et al.* Fatty acids, eicosanoids, and hypolipidemic agents identified as ligands of peroxisome proliferator-activated receptors by coactivator-dependent receptor ligand assay. *Mol. Endocrinol.* **11** (1997) 779-791.

[9]   J.M. Keller, P. Collet, A. Bianchi *et al.* Implications of peroxisome proliferator-activated receptors (PPARS) in development, cell life status and disease. *Int. J. Dev. Biol.* **44** (2000) 429-442.

[10]   P. Escher, O. Braissant, S. Basu-Modak *et al.* Rat PPARs: quantitative analysis in adult rat tissues and regulation in fasting and refeeding. *Endocrinology* **142** (2001) 4195-4202.

[11]   O. Braissant, F. Foufelle, C. Scotto *et al.* Differential expression of peroxisome proliferator-activated receptors (PPARs): tissue distribution of PPAR-alpha, -beta, and -gamma in the adult rat. *Endocrinology* **137** (1996) 354-366.

[12]   D. Auboeuf, J. Rieusset, L. Fajas *et al.* Tissue distribution and quantification of the expression of mRNAs of peroxisome proliferator-activated receptors and liver X receptor-alpha in humans: no alteration in adipose tissue of obese and NIDDM patients. *Diabetes* **46** (1997) 1319-1327.

[13]   R. Mukherjee, L. Jow, G.E. Croston *et al.* Identification, characterization, and tissue distribution of human peroxisome proliferator-activated receptor (PPAR) isoforms PPARgamma2 versus PPARgamma1 and activation with retinoid X receptor agonists and antagonists. *J. Biol. Chem.* **272** (1997) 8071-8076.

[14]   C.N. Palmer, M.H. Hsu, K.J. Griffin *et al.* Peroxisome proliferator activated receptor-alpha expression in human liver. *Mol. Pharmacol.* **53** (1998) 14-22.

[15]   E.D. Rosen and B.M. Spiegelman. PPARgamma: a nuclear regulator of metabolism, differentiation, and cell growth. *J. Biol. Chem.* **276** (2001) 37731-37734.

[16]   Y. Barak, M.C. Nelson, E.S. Ong *et al.* PPAR gamma is required for placental, cardiac, and adipose tissue development. *Mol. Cell* **4** (1999) 585-595.

[17]   O. Braissant and W. Wahli. Differential expression of peroxisome proliferator-activated receptor-alpha, -beta, and -gamma during rat embryonic development. *Endocrinology* **139** (1998) 2748-2754.

[18]   T.E. Cullingford, K. Bhakoo, S. Peuchen *et al.* Distribution of mRNAs encoding the peroxisome proliferator-activated receptor alpha, beta, and gamma and the retinoid X receptor alpha, beta, and gamma in rat central nervous system. *J. Neurochem.* **70** (1998) 1366-1375.

[19]   S. Basu-Modak, O. Braissant, P. Escher *et al.* Peroxisome proliferator-activated receptor beta regulates acyl-CoA synthetase 2 in reaggregated rat brain cell cultures. *J. Biol. Chem.* **274** (1999) 35881-35888.

[20]   J.M. Peters, S.S. Lee, W. Li *et al.* Growth, adipose, brain, and skin alterations resulting from targeted disruption of the mouse peroxisome proliferator-activated receptor beta(delta). *Mol. Cell. Biol.* **20** (2000) 5119-5128.

[21]   A. Cimini, L. Cristiano, S. Colafarina *et al.* PPARgamma-dependent effects of conjugated linoleic acid on the human glioblastoma cell line (ADF). *Int. J. Cancer* **117** (2005) 923-933.

[22]   M.T. Heneka, T. Klockgether, D.L. Feinstein. Peroxisome proliferator-activated receptor-gamma ligands reduce neuronal inducible nitric oxide synthase expression and cell death in vivo. *J. Neurosci.* **20** (2000) 6862-6867. Erratum in: *J. Neurosci.* **20** (2000) 1a.

[23] N.C. Inestrosa, J.A. Godoy, R.A. Quintanilla *et al.* Peroxisome proliferator-activated receptor gamma is expressed in hippocampal neurons and its activation prevents beta-amyloid neurodegeneration: role of Wnt signaling. *Exp. Cell Res.* **304** (2005) 91-104.

[24] K.S. Park, R.D. Lee, S.K. Kang *et al.* Neuronal differentiation of embryonic midbrain cells by upregulation of peroxisome proliferator-activated receptor-gamma via the JNK-dependent pathway. *Exp. Cell Res.* **297** (2004) 424-433.

[25] S.A. Smith, G.R. Monteith, J.A. Robinson *et al.* Effect of the peroxisome proliferator-activated receptor beta activator GW0742 in rat cultured cerebellar granule neurons. *J. Neurosci. Res.* **77** (2004) 240-249.

[26] S. Moreno, S. Farioli-Vecchioli, M.P. Ceru. Immunolocalization of peroxisome proliferator-activated receptors and retinoid X receptors in the adult rat CNS. *Neuroscience* **123** (2004) 131-145.

[27] J.W. Woods, M. Tanen, D.J. Figueroa *et al.* Localization of PPARdelta in murine central nervous system: expression in oligodendrocytes and neurons. *Brain Res.* **975** (2003) 10-21.

[28] A. Cimini, A. Bernardo, M.G. Cifone *et al.* TNFalpha downregulates PPARdelta expression in oligodendrocyte progenitor cells: implications for demyelinating diseases. *Glia* **41** (2003) 3-14. Erratum in: *Glia* **41** (2003) 212.

[29] I. Saluja, J.G. Granneman, R.P. Skoff. PPAR delta agonists stimulate oligodendrocyte differentiation in tissue culture. *Glia* **33** (2001) 191-204.

[30] L. Cristiano, A. Bernardo, M.P. Ceru. Peroxisome proliferator-activated receptors (PPARs) and peroxisomes in rat cortical and cerebellar astrocytes. *J. Neurocytol.* **30** (2001) 671-683.

[31] S. Farioli-Vecchioli, S. Moreno, M.P. Ceru. Immunocytochemical localization of acyl-CoA oxidase in the rat central nervous system. *J. Neurocytol.* **30** (2001) 21-33.

[32] R. Martin, H.F. McFarland, D.E. McFarlin. Immunological aspects of demyelinating diseases. *Annu. Rev. Immunol.* **10** (1992) 153-187.

[33] P.R. Colville-Nash, S.S. Qureshi, D. Willis *et al.* Inhibition of inducible nitric oxide synthase by peroxisome proliferator-activated receptor agonists: correlation with induction of heme oxygenase 1. *J. Immunol.* **161** (1998) 978-984.

[34] C. Jiang, A.T. Ting, B. Seed. PPAR-gamma agonists inhibit production of monocyte inflammatory cytokines. *Nature* **391** (1998) 82-86.

[35] M. Ricote, A.C. Li, T.M. Willson *et al.* The peroxisome proliferator-activated receptor-gamma is a negative regulator of macrophage activation. *Nature* **391** (1998) 79-82.

[36] C.G. Su, X. Wen, S.T. Bailey *et al.* A novel therapy for colitis utilizing PPAR-gamma ligands to inhibit the epithelial inflammatory response. *J. Clin. Invest.* **104** (1999) 383-389.

[37] P. Desreumaux, L. Dubuquoy, S. Nutten *et al.* Attenuation of colon inflammation through activators of the retinoid X receptor (RXR)/peroxisome proliferator-activated receptor gamma (PPARgamma) heterodimer. A basis for new therapeutic strategies. *J. Exp. Med.* **193** (2001) 827-838.

[38] Y. Kawahito, M. Kondo, Y. Tsubouchi *et al.* 15-deoxy-Delta(12,14)-PGJ(2) induces synoviocyte apoptosis and suppresses adjuvant-induced arthritis in rats. *J. Clin. Invest.* **106** (2000) 189-197.

[39] A. Diab, C. Deng, J.D. Smith *et al.* Peroxisome proliferator-activated receptor-gamma agonist 15-deoxy-Delta(12,14)-prostaglandin J(2) ameliorates experimental autoimmune encephalomyelitis. *J. Immunol.* **168** (2002) 2508-2515.

[40] M. Niino, K. Iwabuchi, S. Kikuchi *et al.* Amelioration of experimental autoimmune encephalomyelitis in C57BL/6 mice by an agonist of peroxisome proliferator-activated receptor-gamma. *J. Neuroimmunol.* **116** (2001) 40-48.

[41] D.L. Feinstein, E. Galea, V. Gavrilyuk *et al.* Peroxisome proliferator-activated receptor-gamma agonists prevent experimental autoimmune encephalomyelitis. *Ann. Neurol.* **51** (2002) 694-702.

[42] I.F. Charo and R.M. Ransohoff. The many roles of chemokines and chemokine receptors in inflammation. *N. Engl. J. Med.* **354** (2006) 610-621.

[43] U. Kintscher, S. Goetze, S. Wakino *et al.* Peroxisome proliferator-activated receptor and retinoid X receptor ligands inhibit monocyte chemotactic protein-1-directed migration of monocytes. *Eur. J. Pharmacol.* **401** (2000) 259-270.

[44] N. Marx, F. Mach, A. Sauty *et al.* Peroxisome proliferator-activated receptor-gamma activators inhibit IFN-gamma-induced expression of the T cell-active CXC chemokines IP-10, Mig, and I-TAC in human endothelial cells. *J. Immunol.* **164** (2000) 6503-6508.

[45] A. Chawla, Y. Barak, L. Nagy *et al.* PPAR-gamma dependent and independent effects on macrophage-gene expression in lipid metabolism and inflammation. *Nat. Med.* **7** (2001) 48-52. Comment in: *Nat. Med.* **7** (2001) 23-24.

[46] C. Natarajan, G. Muthian, Y. Barak *et al.* Peroxisome proliferator-activated receptor-gamma-deficient heterozygous mice develop an exacerbated neural antigen-induced Th1 response and experimental allergic encephalomyelitis. *J. Immunol.* **171** (2003) 5743-5750. Erratum in: *J. Immunol.* **172** (2004) following 5127.

[47] H.P. Raikwar, G. Muthian, J. Rajasingh *et al.* PPARgamma antagonists reverse the inhibition of neural antigen-specific Th1 response and experimental allergic encephalomyelitis by Ciglitazone and 15-deoxy-Delta12,14-Prostaglandin J2. *J. Neuroimmunol.* **178** (2006) 76-86.

[48] P. Rieckmann, M. Albrecht, B. Kitze *et al.* Tumor-necrosis-factor-alpha messenger RNA expression in patients with relapsing-remitting multiple sclerosis is associated with disease activity. *Ann. Neurol.* **37** (1995) 82-88.

[49] S. Schmidt, E. Moric, M. Schmidt *et al.* Anti-inflammatory and antiproliferative actions of PPAR-gamma agonists on T lymphocytes derived from MS patients. *J. Leukoc. Biol.* **75** (2004) 478-485.

[50] L. Klotz, M. Schmidt, T. Giese *et al.* Proinflammatory stimulation and pioglitazone treatment regulate peroxisome proliferator-activated receptor gamma levels in peripheral blood mononuclear cells from healthy controls and multiple sclerosis patients. *J. Immunol.* **175** (2005) 4948-4955.

[51] J.M. Gimble, C.E. Robinson, X. Wu *et al.* Peroxisome proliferator-activated receptor-gamma activation by thiazolidinediones induces adipogenesis in bone marrow stromal cells. *Mol. Pharmacol.* **50** (1996) 1087-1094.

[52] M. Kudo, A. Sugawara, A. Uruno *et al.* Transcription suppression of peroxisome proliferator-activated receptor gamma2 gene expression by tumor necrosis factor alpha via an inhibition of CCAAT/enhancer-binding protein delta during the early stage of adipocyte differentiation. *Endocrinology* **145** (2004) 4948-4956.

[53] K.J. Waite, Z.E. Floyd, P. Arbour-Reily *et al.* Interferon-gamma-induced regulation of peroxisome proliferator-activated receptor gamma and STATs in adipocytes. *J. Biol. Chem.* **276** (2001) 7062-7068.

[54] H.A. Pershadsingh. Peroxisome proliferator-activated receptor-gamma: therapeutic target for diseases beyond diabetes: quo vadis? *Expert Opin. Investig. Drugs* **13** (2004) 215-228.

[55] M.T. Heneka, G.E. Landreth, D.L. Feinstein. Role for peroxisome proliferator-activated receptor-gamma in Alzheimer's disease. *Ann. Neurol.* **49** (2001) 276.

[56] B.A. in 't Veld, A. Ruitenberg, A. Hofman *et al.* Nonsteroidal antiinflammatory drugs and the risk of Alzheimer's disease. *N. Engl. J. Med.* **345** (2001) 1515-1521.

[57] T. Kielian and P.D. Drew. Effects of peroxisome proliferator-activated receptor-gamma agonists on central nervous system inflammation. *J. Neurosci. Res.* **71** (2003) 315-325.

[58] G.E. Landreth and M.T. Heneka. Anti-inflammatory actions of peroxisome proliferator-activated receptor gamma agonists in Alzheimer's disease. *Neurobiol. Aging* **22** (2001) 937-944.

[59] H. Akiyama, S. Barger, S. Barnum *et al.* Inflammation and Alzheimer's disease. *Neurobiol. Aging* **21** (2000) 383-421.

[60] M. Hull, K. Lieb, B.L. Fiebich. Pathways of inflammatory activation in Alzheimer's disease: potential targets for disease modifying drugs. *Curr. Med. Chem.* **9** (2002) 83-88.

[61] M.T. Heneka, H. Wiesinger, L. Dumitrescu-Ozimek *et al.* Neuronal and glial coexpression of argininosuccinate synthetase and inducible nitric oxide synthase in Alzheimer disease. *J. Neuropathol. Exp. Neurol.* **60** (2001) 906-916.

[62] S.C. Lee, M.L. Zhao, A. Hirano *et al.* Inducible nitric oxide synthase immunoreactivity in the Alzheimer disease hippocampus: association with Hirano bodies, neurofibrillary tangles, and senile plaques. *J. Neuropathol. Exp. Neurol.* **58** (1999) 1163-1169.

[63] Y. Vodovotz, M.S. Lucia, K.C. Flanders *et al.* Inducible nitric oxide synthase in tangle-bearing neurons of patients with Alzheimer's disease. *J. Exp. Med.* **184** (1996) 1425-1433.

[64] M.T. Heneka, D.L. Feinstein, E. Galea *et al.* Peroxisome proliferator-activated receptor gamma agonists protect cerebellar granule cells from cytokine-induced apoptotic cell death by inhibition of inducible nitric oxide synthase. *J. Neuroimmunol.* **100** (1999) 156-168.

[65] C.K. Combs, D.E. Johnson, J.C. Karlo *et al.* Inflammatory mechanisms in Alzheimer's disease: inhibition of beta-amyloid-stimulated proinflammatory responses and neurotoxicity by PPARgamma agonists. *J. Neurosci.* **20** (2000) 558-567.

[66] R.A. Daynes and D.C. Jones. Emerging roles of PPARs in inflammation and immunity. *Nat. Rev. Immunol.* **2** (2002) 748-759.

[67] E.J. Kim, K.J. Kwon, J.Y. Park *et al.* Effects of peroxisome proliferator-activated receptor agonists on LPS-induced neuronal death in mixed cortical neurons: associated with iNOS and COX-2. *Brain Res.* **941** (2002) 1-10.

[68] R. Luna-Medina, M. Cortes-Canteli, M. Alonso *et al.* Regulation of inflammatory response in neural cells in vitro by thiadiazolidinones derivatives through peroxisome proliferator-activated receptor gamma activation. *J. Biol. Chem.* **280** (2005) 21453-21462.

[69] M.T. Heneka, V. Gavrilyuk, G.E. Landreth *et al.* Noradrenergic depletion increases inflammatory responses in brain: effects on IkappaB and HSP70 expression. *J. Neurochem.* **85** (2003) 387-398.

[70] Y. Maeshiba, Y. Kiyota, K. Yamashita *et al.* Disposition of the new antidiabetic agent pioglitazone in rats, dogs, and monkeys. *Arzneimittelforschung* **47** (1997) 29-35.

[71] Q. Yan, J. Zhang, H. Liu *et al.* Anti-inflammatory drug therapy alters beta-amyloid processing and deposition in an animal model of Alzheimer's disease. *J. Neurosci.* **23** (2003) 7504-7509.

[72]   M.T. Heneka, M. Sastre, L. Dumitrescu-Ozimek *et al.* Acute treatment with the PPARgamma agonist pioglitazone and ibuprofen reduces glial inflammation and Abeta1-42 levels in APPV717I transgenic mice. *Brain* **128** (2005) 1442-1453.

[73]   M. Sastre, I. Dewachter, G.E. Landreth *et al.* Nonsteroidal anti-inflammatory drugs and peroxisome proliferator-activated receptor-gamma agonists modulate immunostimulated processing of amyloid precursor protein through regulation of beta-secretase. *J. Neurosci.* **23** (2003) 9796-9804.

[74]   M. Sastre, I. Dewachter, S. Rossner *et al.* Nonsteroidal anti-inflammatory drugs repress beta-secretase gene promoter activity by the activation of PPARgamma. *Proc. Natl. Acad. Sci. U.S.A.* **103** (2006) 443-448.

[75]   C. d'Abramo, S. Massone, J.M. Zingg *et al.* Role of peroxisome proliferator-activated receptor gamma in amyloid precursor protein processing and amyloid beta-mediated cell death. *Biochem. J.* **391** (2005) 693-698.

[76]   I.E. Camacho, L. Serneels, K. Spittaels *et al.* Peroxisome-proliferator-activated receptor gamma induces a clearance mechanism for the amyloid-beta peptide. *J. Neurosci.* **24** (2004) 10908-10917.

[77]   W.A. Pedersen, P.J. McMillan, J.J. Kulstad *et al.* Rosiglitazone attenuates learning and memory deficits in Tg2576 Alzheimer mice. *Exp. Neurol.* **199** (2006) 265-273. Comment in: *Exp. Neurol.* **199** (2006) 245-248.

[78]   W.Q. Qiu and M.F. Folstein. Insulin, insulin-degrading enzyme and amyloid-beta peptide in Alzheimer's disease: review and hypothesis. *Neurobiol. Aging* **27** (2006) 190-198.

[79]   M.E. Risner, A.M. Saunders, J.F. Altman *et al.* Efficacy of rosiglitazone in a genetically defined population with mild-to-moderate Alzheimer's disease. *Pharmacogenomics J.* **6** (2006) 246-254. Comment in: *Pharmacogenomics J.* **6** (2006) 222-224.

[80]   G.S. Watson, B.A. Cholerton, M.A. Reger *et al.* Preserved cognition in patients with early Alzheimer disease and amnestic mild cognitive impairment during treatment with rosiglitazone: a preliminary study. *Am. J. Geriatr. Psychiatry* **13** (2005) 950-958.

[81]   M. Chalimoniuk, K. King-Pospisil, W.A. Pedersen *et al.* Arachidonic acid increases choline acetyltransferase activity in spinal cord neurons through a protein kinase C-mediated mechanism. *J. Neurochem.* **90** (2004) 629-636.

[82]   J.A. Luchsinger, M.X. Tang, Y. Stern *et al.* Diabetes mellitus and risk of Alzheimer's disease and dementia with stroke in a multiethnic cohort. *Am. J. Epidemiol.* **154** (2001) 635-641.

[83]   G.S. Watson and S. Craft. The role of insulin resistance in the pathogenesis of Alzheimer's disease: implications for treatment. *CNS Drugs* **17** (2003) 27-45.

[84]   R. Peila, B.L. Rodriguez, L.J. Launer. Type 2 diabetes, APOE gene, and the risk for dementia and related pathologies: The Honolulu-Asia Aging Study. *Diabetes* **51** (2002) 1256-1262.

[85]   D. Geldmacher and G. Landreth. Pioglitazone in Alzheimer's Disease: Rationale and Clinical Trial Design. (2004) 397.

[86]   D.L. Feinstein, A. Spagnolo, C. Akar *et al.* Receptor-independent actions of PPAR thiazolidinedione agonists: is mitochondrial function the key? *Biochem. Pharmacol.* **70** (2005) 177-188.

[87]   W.A. Pedersen and E.R. Flynn. Insulin resistance contributes to aberrant stress responses in the Tg2576 mouse model of Alzheimer's disease. *Neurobiol. Dis.* **17** (2004) 500-506.

[88]   S. Craft, S. Asthana, G. Schellenberg *et al.* Insulin effects on glucose metabolism, memory, and plasma amyloid precursor protein in Alzheimer's disease differ according to apolipoprotein-E genotype. *Ann. N.Y. Acad. Sci.* **903** (2000) 222-228.

[89]   S. Craft, S. Asthana, G. Schellenberg *et al.* Insulin metabolism in Alzheimer's disease differs according to apolipoprotein E genotype and gender. *Neuroendocrinology* **70** (1999) 146-152.

[90]   J. Kuusisto, K. Koivisto, L. Mykkanen *et al.* Association between features of the insulin resistance syndrome and Alzheimer's disease independently of apolipoprotein E4 phenotype: cross sectional population based study. *BMJ* **315** (1997) 1045-1049.

[91]   P. Hantraye, E. Brouillet, R. Ferrante *et al.* Inhibition of neuronal nitric oxide synthase prevents MPTP-induced parkinsonism in baboons. *Nat. Med.* **2** (1996) 1017-1021. Comment in: *Nat. Med.* **2** (1996) 965-966.

[92]   S. Przedborski, V. Jackson-Lewis, R. Yokoyama *et al.* Role of neuronal nitric oxide in 1-methyl-4-phenyl-1,2,3,6-tetrahydropyridine (MPTP)-induced dopaminergic neurotoxicity. *Proc. Natl. Acad. Sci. U.S.A.* **93** (1996) 4565-4571.

[93]   J.B. Schulz, R.T. Matthews, M.M. Muqit *et al.* Inhibition of neuronal nitric oxide synthase by 7-nitroindazole protects against MPTP-induced neurotoxicity in mice. *J. Neurochem.* **64** (1995) 936-939.

[94]   S. Hunot, B. Brugg, D. Ricard *et al.* Nuclear translocation of NF-kappaB is increased in dopaminergic neurons of patients with parkinson disease. *Proc. Natl. Acad. Sci. U.S.A.* **94** (1997) 7531-7536.

[95]   T. Dehmer, J. Lindenau, S. Haid *et al.* Deficiency of inducible nitric oxide synthase protects against MPTP toxicity in vivo. *J. Neurochem.* **74** (2000) 2213-2216.

[96]   G.T. Liberatore, V. Jackson-Lewis, S. Vukosavic *et al.* Inducible nitric oxide synthase stimulates dopaminergic neurodegeneration in the MPTP model of Parkinson disease. *Nat. Med.* **5** (1999) 1403-1409. Comment in: *Nat. Med.* **5** (1999) 1354-1355.

[97]   T. Breidert, J. Callebert, M.T. Heneka *et al.* Protective action of the peroxisome proliferator-activated receptor-gamma agonist pioglitazone in a mouse model of Parkinson's disease. *J. Neurochem.* **82** (2002) 615-624.

[98]   T. Dehmer, M.T. Heneka, M. Sastre *et al.* Protection by pioglitazone in the MPTP model of Parkinson's disease correlates with I kappa B alpha induction and block of NF kappa B and iNOS activation. *J. Neurochem.* **88** (2004) 494-501.

[99]   H. Chen, E. Jacobs, M.A. Schwarzschild *et al.* Nonsteroidal antiinflammatory drug use and the risk for Parkinson's disease. *Ann. Neurol.* **58** (2005) 963-967. Comment in: *Ann. Neurol.* **59** (2006) 988-989.

[100]   H. Chen, S.M. Zhang, M.A. Hernan *et al.* Nonsteroidal anti-inflammatory drugs and the risk of Parkinson disease. *Arch. Neurol.* **60** (2003) 1059-1064. Comment in: *Arch. Neurol.* **60** (2003) 1043-1044.

[101]   J.M. Lehmann, J.M. Lenhard, B.B. Oliver *et al.* Peroxisome proliferator-activated receptors alpha and gamma are activated by indomethacin and other non-steroidal anti-inflammatory drugs. *J. Biol. Chem.* **272** (1997) 3406-3410.

[102]   P.L. McGeer and E.G. McGeer. Inflammatory processes in amyotrophic lateral sclerosis. *Muscle Nerve* **26** (2002) 459-470.

[103]   P. Weydt and T. Moller. Neuroinflammation in the pathogenesis of amyotrophic lateral sclerosis. *Neuroreport* **16** (2005) 527-531.

[104]   M. Kiaei, K. Kipiani, J. Chen *et al.* Peroxisome proliferator-activated receptor-gamma agonist extends survival in transgenic mouse model of amyotrophic lateral sclerosis. *Exp. Neurol.* **191** (2005) 331-336.

[105]   B. Schutz, J. Reimann, L. Dumitrescu-Ozimek *et al.* The oral antidiabetic pioglitazone protects from neurodegeneration and amyotrophic lateral sclerosis-like symptoms in superoxide dismutase-G93A transgenic mice. *J. Neurosci.* **25** (2005) 7805-7812.

[106]   F.C. Barone, L.M. Hillegass, M.N. Tzimas *et al.* Time-related changes in myeloperoxidase activity and leukotriene B4 receptor binding reflect leukocyte influx in cerebral focal stroke. *Mol. Chem. Neuropathol.* **24** (1995) 13-30.

[107]   F.C. Barone and G.Z. Feuerstein. Inflammatory mediators and stroke: new opportunities for novel therapeutics. *J. Cereb. Blood Flow Metab.* **19** (1999) 819-834.

[108]   K.J. Becker. Inflammation and acute stroke. *Curr. Opin. Neurol.* **11** (1998) 45-49.

[109]   Z. Zheng and M.A. Yenari. Post-ischemic inflammation: molecular mechanisms and therapeutic implications. *Neurol. Res.* **26** (2004) 884-892.

[110]   M. Chopp, Y. Li, N. Jiang *et al.* Antibodies against adhesion molecules reduce apoptosis after transient middle cerebral artery occlusion in rat brain. *J. Cereb. Blood Flow Metab.* **16** (1996) 578-584.

[111]   C. Iadecola and M.E. Ross. Molecular pathology of cerebral ischemia: delayed gene expression and strategies for neuroprotection. *Ann. N.Y. Acad. Sci.* **835** (1997) 203-217.

[112]   J.K. Relton and N.J. Rothwell. Interleukin-1 receptor antagonist inhibits ischaemic and excitotoxic neuronal damage in the rat. *Brain Res. Bull.* **29** (1992) 243-246.

[113]   G.Y. Yang, C. Gong, Z. Qin *et al.* Inhibition of TNFalpha attenuates infarct volume and ICAM-1 expression in ischemic mouse brain. *Neuroreport* **9** (1998) 2131-2134.

[114]   R.L. Zhang, M. Chopp, Y. Li *et al.* Anti-ICAM-1 antibody reduces ischemic cell damage after transient middle cerebral artery occlusion in the rat. *Neurology* **44** (1994) 1747-1751.

[115]   S. Sundararajan and G.E. Landreth. Antiinflammatory properties of PPARgamma agonists following ischemia. *Drug News Perspect.* **17** (2004) 229-236.

[116]   S. Sundararajan, J.L. Gamboa, N.A. Victor *et al.* Peroxisome proliferator-activated receptor-gamma ligands reduce inflammation and infarction size in transient focal ischemia. *Neuroscience* **130** (2005) 685-696.

[117]   N.A. Victor, E.W. Wanderi, J. Gamboa *et al.* Altered PPARgamma expression and activation after transient focal ischemia in rats. *Eur. J. Neurosci.* **24** (2006) 1653-1663.

[118]   T. Shimazu, I. Inoue, N. Araki *et al.* A peroxisome proliferator-activated receptor-gamma agonist reduces infarct size in transient but not in permanent ischemia. *Stroke* **36** (2005) 353-359.

[119]   Y. Zhao, A. Patzer, P. Gohlke *et al.* The intracerebral application of the PPARgamma-ligand pioglitazone confers neuroprotection against focal ischaemia in the rat brain. *Eur. J. Neurosci.* **22** (2005) 278-282.

[120]   M.P. Pereira, O. Hurtado, A. Cardenas *et al.* The nonthiazolidinedione PPARgamma agonist L-796,449 is neuroprotective in experimental stroke. *J. Neuropathol. Exp. Neurol.* **64** (2005) 797-805.

[121]   M. Allahtavakoli, A.P. Shabanzadeh, S.S. Sadr *et al.* Rosiglitazone, a peroxisome proliferator-activated receptor-gamma ligand, reduces infarction volume and neurological deficits in an embolic model of stroke. *Clin. Exp. Pharmacol. Physiol.* **33** (2006) 1052-1058.

[122] M. Collino, M. Aragno, R. Mastrocola *et al.* Modulation of the oxidative stress and inflammatory response by PPAR-gamma agonists in the hippocampus of rats exposed to cerebral ischemia/reperfusion. *Eur. J. Pharmacol.* **530** (2006) 70-80.

[123] Y. Luo, W. Yin, A.P. Signore *et al.* Neuroprotection against focal ischemic brain injury by the peroxisome proliferator-activated receptor-gamma agonist rosiglitazone. *J. Neurochem.* **97** (2006) 435-448.

[124] M.P. Pereira, O. Hurtado, A. Cardenas *et al.* Rosiglitazone and 15-deoxy-Delta12,14-prostaglandin J2 cause potent neuroprotection after experimental stroke through noncompletely overlapping mechanisms. *J. Cereb. Blood Flow Metab.* **26** (2006) 218-229.

[125] D. Deplanque, P. Gele, O. Petrault *et al.* Peroxisome proliferator-activated receptor-alpha activation as a mechanism of preventive neuroprotection induced by chronic fenofibrate treatment. *J. Neurosci.* **23** (2003) 6264-6271.

[126] M. Collino, M. Aragno, R. Mastrocola *et al.* Oxidative stress and inflammatory response evoked by transient cerebral ischemia/reperfusion: effects of the PPAR-alpha agonist WY14643. *Free Radic. Biol. Med.* **41** (2006) 579-589. Erratum in: *Free Radic. Biol. Med.* **41** (2006) 1619.

[127] D. Arsenijevic, F. de Bilbao, J. Plamondon *et al.* Increased infarct size and lack of hyperphagic response after focal cerebral ischemia in peroxisome proliferator-activated receptor beta-deficient mice. *J. Cereb. Blood Flow Metab.* **26** (2006) 433-435.

[128] J.A. Dormandy, B. Charbonnel, D.J. Eckland *et al.* Secondary prevention of macrovascular events in patients with type 2 diabetes in the PROactive Study (PROspective pioglitAzone Clinical Trial In macroVascular Events): a randomised controlled trial. *Lancet* **366** (2005) 1279-1289.

[129] J. Lee and M. Reding. Effects of thiazolidinediones on stroke recovery: a case-matched controlled study. *Neurochem. Res.* **32** (2007) 635-638.

[130] B.C. Lee, H.J. Lee, J.H. Chung. Peroxisome proliferator-activated receptor-gamma2 Pro12Ala polymorphism is associated with reduced risk for ischemic stroke with type 2 diabetes. *Neurosci. Lett.* **410** (2006) 141-145.

Molecular Biology of Circadian Rhythms and Cardiometabolic Disease: Role of the Orphan Nuclear Receptor Rev-erbα

Bart Staels and Hélène Duez
Inserm U.545, Institut Pasteur de Lille, 1 rue du Professeur Calmette, BP 245, 59019 Lille, France; and Université de Lille 2, Lille, 59006 France

Abstract. Circadian patterns of cardiovascular vulnerability have been well documented, with a peak incidence of cardiovascular events in the morning. Recent studies have outlined the importance of the "Clock genes" in the development of metabolic disorders predisposing to atherosclerosis. Rev-erbα is a nuclear receptor that regulates hepatic and adipose lipid metabolism as well as vascular inflammation. Recent findings identify Rev-erbα also as a major regulator of the circadian regulation of metabolic pathways. Moreover, cross-talk between Rev-erbα and other nuclear receptors well described as key regulators of atherosclerosis may converge to integrate metabolic and circadian signals.

Keywords. Circadian rhythm, cardiovascular disease, metabolic syndrome, Rev-erbα, Nuclear Receptors

Abbreviations

cardiovascular disease (CVD), nuclear receptor (NR), suprachiasmatic nucleus (SCN), cryptochrome (Cry), period (Per), thyroid receptor (TR), RAR-related orphan receptor (ROR), endothelial cells (ECs), vascular smooth muscle cells (VSMCs), interleukin (IL), tumor necrosis factor (TNF), nuclear factor κB (NFκB), cycloxygenase (COX), staggerer (sg/sg), plasminogen activator inhibitor 1 (PAI-1), apolipoprotein (Apo), peroxisome proliferator-activated receptor (PPAR), CCAAT/enhancer-binding protein (C/EBP), differentiation-dependent factor 1/sterol regulatory element-binding protein (ADD-1/SREBP-1).

Introduction

In mammals, including humans, many physiological processes are under the control of day-night rhythms. Hormone secretion, lipid and carbohydrate metabolism, feeding behaviour and blood pressure are some examples of processes subject to daily variations [1]. As a consequence, many diseases display symptoms and onset characteristics which are not randomly distributed within a 24 hours period. In particular, circadian patterns of cardiovascular vulnerability have been well documented, with a peak incidence of cardiovascular events such as myocardial infarction, sudden cardiac death and stroke higher early in the morning than in other day times [2,3]. Epidemiological and pathophysiological studies also indicate a causal link between disrupted biological timing and the metabolic syndrome, which is associated with an increased risk of accelerated atherosclerosis and cardiovascular disease (CVD) [4]. The metabolic syndrome describes a complex of metabolic abnormalities, including obesity, diabetes, hypertension, and dyslipidemia, in which insulin resistance is central.

Molecular mechanism of circadian rhythmicity is modelled by a transcription/translation feedback oscillator in which Rev-erbα has been identified as a critical regulator and target of the Clock genes [5]. Rev-erbα is a member of the nuclear receptor (NR) superfamily. Although its biological function remains largely unknown, Rev-erbα has been implicated in lipid metabolism, adipogenesis and vascular inflammation [6-9]. This review discusses the scientific rationale behind circadian cycling and CVD events/risks and examines the contribution of Rev-erbα as a molecular integrator between these biological pathways.

Rev-erbα: A Critical Regulator and Target of the Clock Genes

Circadian rhythms are generated by a pacemaker located in the suprachiasmatic nucleus (SCN) of the hypothalamus. Light acts as the primary stimulus to synchronise the internal clock with the environment. Specialised cells of the retina detect the light and transmit information along the retinohypothalamic nerve tract to the SCN. In addition, circadian oscillators have been described in many peripheral tissues such as liver, adipose tissue and heart with different phases from those observed in the SCN.

The central component of the circadian period is a molecular oscillator generated by autoregulatory feedback loops of Clock gene expression. In mammals, Bmal1 and Clock activate transcription of the cryptochrome (Cry) and period (Per). Once the Per and Cry proteins have reached a critical concentration, they inhibit their own synthesis through post-translational regulation [10]. Rev-erbα transcription is activated by Bmal1-Clock heterodimer and inhibited by Cry and Per proteins resulting in oscillation of the Rev-erbα gene expression. In turn, Rev-erbα represses Bmal1 and also Clock gene expression, so linking the positive and negative limbs of the feedback loops [5].

Rev-erbα deficient mice present a drastic reduction of circadian rhythms in the transcription of Clock and Bmal1, whereas no arrhythmic behaviour was observed when mice are placed in a constant environment [5]. However, Rev-erbα knock-out mice display a significantly shorter period length than wild-type animals. Interestingly, transgenic mice expressing multiple Clock gene copies show a similar phenotype [11]. So, even if Rev-erbα is not required for basic oscillator function, it is critical for the robustness of the oscillation and the resynchronisation of the circadian timing [5].

Rev-erbα: An Atypical Nuclear Receptor

The NR superfamily is composed of transcription factors that have emerged as key regulators of metabolism, inflammation and cell differentiation. In addition to the well-known ligand-activated NRs, several members within this superfamily, such as Rev-erbs, have no identified ligand and are referred to as « orphan NRs ». The Rev-erb subfamily contains two members: Rev-erbα (NR1D1) [12] and Rev-erbβ (NR1D2) [13]. Both mouse and human homologues of Rev-erbα are encoded on the opposite strand of the thyroid receptor (TR) α gene, that encodes TRα1 and its splice variant TRα2 [12]. Rev-erbα and TRα2 mRNA products have a 269 nucleotides overlap and Rev-erbα mRNA inhibits the splicing reaction that generates TRα2 *in vitro* [14]. Rev-erbα is highly expressed in adipose tissue, skeletal muscle, brain and liver and its expression is induced during adipocyte differentiation [12]. Onishi *et al* have shown that Rev-erbα displays circadian expression profile in the SCN of mouse brain [15]. In addition, in rat liver as well as in cultured human primary hepatocytes and rat fibroblasts Rev-erbα expression oscillates with a circadian rhythm [16,17]. Recently, it has also been described a robust circadian expression of Rev-erbα in murine brown, inguinal, and epididymal adipose tissues [18].

Molecular modelling of the putative ligand-binding domain of Rev-erbα suggests that the ligand pocket is occupied by amino-acid side chains and that the small residual cavity is unlikely to bind a classical ligand [19]. Therefore, regulation of Rev-erbα expression and/or post-translational modifications constitutes a crucial step for this receptor activity control. Notably, phosphorylation of Rev-erbα protein stabilizes its expression and thus is an important level of control of its activity [20]. Moreover, Rev-erbα and β are the only members in the NR family that lacks the AF-2 domain and according to modelling studies; Rev-erbs have revealed a very hydrophobic surface due to the absence of helix 12 via which co-repressors are recruited. As a consequence, Rev-erbs act as negative regulators of transcription after binding either as a monomer to a response element composed of the consensus half-site motif (A/G)GGTCA preceded by an A/T rich 5' sequence (RevRE), or as a homodimer to a direct repeat of the core motif spaced by two nucleotides (Rev-DR2) [21]. Other closely related nuclear receptors, RAR-related orphan receptors (ROR) bind to the same response elements, but have opposite effects on transcription [13]. Interestingly, RORα activates Rev-erbα transcription [22] and Rev-erbα represses its own expression [23] binding on the same site.

Rev-erbα: An Integrator between Cardiovascular Disease Events and Circadian Rhythmicity

Atherosclerosis, the main origin of CVD, is a long-term chronic disease characterized by the accumulation of lipids and fibrous connective tissue in the large arteries, accompanied by a local inflammatory response [24]. Under basal conditions, the endothelium forms a relatively impermeable barrier between the circulating blood and the vessel wall. Endothelial injury is thought to be the primary event in atherosclerosis which leads to the attraction, recruitment and activation of different cell-types, including monocytes/macrophages, T-lymphocytes, endothelial cells (ECs) and vascular smooth muscle cells (VSMCs). The activation of these cells leads to the release of pro-inflammatory molecules, such as cytokines, and the onset of a chronic inflammatory response. Rev-erbα is expressed in ECs and VSMCs [6] and its expression has been recently reported in murine bone marrow-derived macrophages and in human peripheral blood mononuclear cells [25,26].

An important occurrence in patients with acute myocardial infarction is the recruitment and the activation of leukocytes in the injured tissue [24]. Both immune cell number and immune functions vary during the 24-h circadian period [27]. Indeed, the nocturnal peak of inflammatory activity such as interleukin (IL)-6 expression could be associated with a greater incidence of CVD risk, possibly causing inflammation of the atherosclerotic plaques and favouring the triggering of an acute coronary syndrome. Migita *et al* have shown that Rev-erbα potentiates the tumor necrosis factor (TNF)α-induced nuclear factor (NF)-κB activation in VSMCs [6]. In these cells, transient over-expression of

Rev-erbα up-regulated inflammatory markers gene expression (e.g. IL-6 and Cycloxygenase(COX)-2)) via induction of NFκB nucleus translocation. RORα is also expressed in vascular cells, where it suppresses TNFα-induced expression of pro-inflammatory genes such as IL-6 and COX2 [28-30].

In addition, the biological effects of cytokines have been shown to change during the light/dark cycle due to changes in physiological cortisol levels [31]. Interestingly, Rev-erbα expression was previously shown to be down-regulated by glucocorticoids [16]. In addition, mice treated with a synthetic glucocorticoid, prednisolone display repressed Rev-erbα and Bmal1 expression [32]. The staggerer (sg/sg) mutant mouse, homozygous for a deletion in the RORα gene, overproduces inflammatory cytokines and lacks the diurnal shift in corticosterone levels [33]. This feature might be related the role of RORα in the regulation of circadian rhythm in SCN. Indeed, as previously shown for Rev-erbα, RORα regulates Bmal1 expression [34]. The competing activities of Rev-erbs and RORs on the same promoter element drive the rhythm in Bmal1 transcription [35]. Cross-talk between Rev-erbα and RORα activities may thus integrate the circadian rhythm regulation of cortisol secretion and the inflammatory response.

The morning excess of cardiac events may also result from a natural circadian variation in fibrinolytic activity. Plasminogen activator inhibitor 1 (PAI-1) is a major inhibitor of fibrinolysis and several lines of evidence suggest that elevated PAI-1 may indeed promote the development of atherothrombosis [36]. PAI-1 exhibits a diurnal pattern in its expression and regulation of its expression by Rev-erbα therefore represents a novel role of this NR as an integrator between the circadian clock and CVD [37]. Interestingly, PAI-1 regulation by Rev-erbα is another example in which Rev-erbα acts by blocking RORα-mediated activation [37].

Rev-erbα: A Link between Transcription Factors of the Clock Machinery and Nuclear Receptors Controlling Metabolism

In addition to cardiovascular events, many risks predisposing to CVD are controlled by circadian rhytmicity. Dysregulation of metabolic pathways, such as metabolism of glucose, cholesterol and fatty acids results in the development of dyslipidemia, insulin resistance, obesity and hypertension. These disorders often occur simultaneously and have therefore been grouped under the term "metabolic syndrome", which is associated with an increased risk of accelerated atherosclerosis and CVD.

Clock genes show patterns of rhythmic expression in peripheral organs, such as liver and adipose tissue [18,38], two organs in which Rev-erbα is highly expressed. Indeed, it has been recently shown a robust and coordinated expression of circadian oscillator genes in murine brown, inguinal, and epididymal adipose tissues [18]. These rhythms correlate with respective gene expression in liver and with the serum markers of circadian function. In obese and diabetics animals, the rhythmic expression of adipocytokines that control energy homeostasis, glucose and lipid metabolism are disturbed [39].

The presence of circadian oscillator genes has significant metabolic implications, and their characterization may have potential therapeutic relevance with respect to the pathogenesis and treatment of the metabolic syndrome [4]. Indeed, it has been demonstrated that an animal model with a known circadian dysregulation displays metabolic problems [40-42]. Turek *et al* have shown that mice homozygous for a loss-of-function mutation in the Clock gene have altered patterns of food intake: they eat too much, become obese and develop metabolic syndrome metabolic syndrome features such as of hyperleptinemia, hyperlipidemia, hepatic steatosis, hyperglycemia, and hypoinsulinemia.

Similar observations have been obtained with Bmal1 [41]. Indeed, Rudic *et al* have found that mutations in Bmal1 and Clock not only modified the diurnal variation in levels of plasma glucose and triglycerides, but also influenced the development of glucose intolerance and insulin resistance in response to a high-fat diet [43]. A central issue is now to identify and understand the molecular mechanism that link master Clock genes such as Clock and Bmal1 to metabolic outputs.

Interestingly, besides its role in circadian regulation, Rev-erbα has also been implicated in the control of several aspects of lipid homeostasis such as lipoprotein metabolism and adipocyte differentiation. ApoC-III gene expression, a major constituent of triglyceride-rich remnant lipoproteins, is repressed by Rev-erbα [7]. Elevated serum levels of triglyceride-rich remnant lipoproteins are a major risk factor predisposing a subject to atherosclerosis. In agreement with these observations Rev-erbα null mice possess elevated levels of ApoC-III expression in serum and liver as well as elevated triglyceride levels [7]. It is interesting to note that plasma triglyceride and ApoC-III protein concentrations in sg/sg mice were significantly lower than in wild-type littermates [44]. This is a new illustration of opposite effect between RORα and Rev-erbα. Rev-erbα has been also involved in repressing rodent ApoA1 gene expression [45], another RORα target gene [46]. *In vivo* studies have shown that ApoA1 reduces free cholesterol accumulation in atherosclerotic lesions of ApoE-deficient mice [47].

In addition, hypolipidemic fibrate drugs induce Rev-erbα mRNA expression [48] via peroxisome proliferator-activated receptor (PPAR)α activation in human liver. PPARs are lipid-activated factors that regulate lipid and lipoprotein metabolism, glucose homeostasis and inflammation, major risk factors for atherosclerosis. The PPAR subfamily consists of three distinct subtypes: PPARα, implicated in fatty acid metabolism, PPARγ, a key factor involved in adipogenesis and PPARβ/δ, whose role is beginning to be understood. In addition to their beneficial effects on metabolic disorders, PPARα and PPARγ also decrease atherosclerosis progression by directly acting at the level on the vascular wall. These both PPAR isoforms induce Rev-erbα expression respectively in liver and adipose tissue [8,48]. As previously described for ROR and Rev-erb family, there is a cross-talk between Rev-erb and PPAR nuclear receptors, which is governed by two mechanisms. On the one hand, Rev-erbα could mediate PPAR action. Therefore, genes regulated by Rev-erbα such as rat ApoA-I [45], will be negatively regulated by PPARα via an indirect mechanism. In addition, adipocyte differentiation is promoted by ectopic Rev-erbα expression in 3T3-L1 cell line, especially in cells treated with the PPARγ ligand, rosiglitazone. Expression of Rev-erbα increases the expression of PPARγ target genes aP2 and CCAAT/enhancer-binding protein (C/EBP)α, but has no effect on C/EBPβ or differentiation-dependent factor 1/sterol regulatory element-binding protein (ADD-1/SREBP-1) gene expression. This suggests a role for Rev-erbα as an enhancer of adipogenesis acting downstream of PPARγ [8]. On the other hand, PPARs and Rev-erbα may compete for binding to similar sites. Indeed, Rev-erbα acts as a negative regulator of the peroxisome proliferator-activated receptor (PPAR)α dependent transactivation by inhibiting expression of the hydratase-dehydrogenase gene [49] and the microsomal cytochrome P450 fatty acid ω-hydroxylase [50], two enzymes implicated in the hepatic peroxisomal fatty acid beta-oxidation [34]. Moreover PPARα and PPARγ interfere with the negative autoregulatory loop of Rev-erbα expression via the Rev-DR2 site.

Finally, there is growing evidence that melatonin, one of the endocrine output signals of the circadian clock, can influence CVD risks. Melatonin provides the organism with circadian information and can be considered as an endogenous synchronizer, able to stabilize and reinforce circadian rhythm. This pineal hormone regulate important processes linked to CVD such as glucose metabolism [51], oxidative stress [52] and blood pressure

[53]. Recent observations indicate that melatonin induces an immediate phase advance of the Rev-erbα rhythm. Rev-erbα may thus be initial molecular targets involved in the chronobiotic effect of melatonin [54]. Interestingly, it was previously described that the effects of melatonin on transcriptional regulation depend on the expression of ROR and support the concept that the receptor is a mediator of nuclear melatonin signalling [55]. These findings illustrate a new example via which NRs and in particular Rev-erbα and RORα could link biology of the circadian rhythm and CVD.

Conclusion

Rev-erbα is an integral component of the complex transcriptional machinery that governs circadian rhythmcity. In addition, Rev-erbα appears to drive transcriptional feedback loops of many NRs (e.g. RORs, PPARs) leading to metabolic flexibility in the control of lipid metabolism, thrombosis and inflammation. These findings collectively lead to the concept that Rev-erbα may establish a molecular link between the clock system and CVD.

References

[1]   F. Gachon, E. Nagoshi, S.A. Brown *et al.* The mammalian circadian timing system: from gene expression to physiology. *Chromosoma* **113** (2004) 103-112.

[2]   J.E. Muller, P.L. Ludmer, S.N. Willich *et al.* Circadian variation in the frequency of sudden cardiac death. *Circulation* **75** (1987) 131-138.

[3]   J.E. Muller, P.H. Stone, Z.G. Turi *et al.* Circadian variation in the frequency of onset of acute myocardial infarction. *N. Engl. J. Med.* **313** (1985) 1315-1322.

[4]   B. Staels. When the Clock stops ticking, metabolic syndrome explodes. *Nat. Med.* **12** (2006) 54-55; discussion 55.

[5]   N. Preitner, F. Damiola, L. Lopez-Molina *et al.* The orphan nuclear receptor REV-ERBalpha controls circadian transcription within the positive limb of the mammalian circadian oscillator. *Cell* **110** (2002) 251-260.

[6]   H. Migita, J. Morser, K. Kawai. Rev-erbalpha upregulates NF-kappaB-responsive genes in vascular smooth muscle cells. *FEBS Lett.* **561** (2004) 69-74.

[7]   E. Raspe, H. Duez, A. Mansen *et al.* Identification of Rev-erbalpha as a physiological repressor of apoC-III gene transcription. *J. Lipid Res.* **43** (2002) 2172-2179.

[8]   C. Fontaine, G. Dubois, Y. Duguay *et al.* The orphan nuclear receptor Rev-Erbalpha is a peroxisome proliferator-activated receptor (PPAR) gamma target gene and promotes PPARgamma-induced adipocyte differentiation. *J. Biol. Chem.* **278** (2003) 37672-37680.

[9]   P. Pircher, P. Chomez, F. Yu *et al.* Aberrant expression of myosin isoforms in skeletal muscles from mice lacking the rev-erbAalpha orphan receptor gene. *Am. J. Physiol. Regul. Integr. Comp. Physiol.* **288** (2005) R482-R490.

[10]   U. Schibler and P. Sassone-Corsi. A web of circadian pacemakers. *Cell* **111** (2002) 919-922.

[11]   M.P. Antoch, E.J. Song, A.M. Chang *et al.* Functional identification of the mouse circadian Clock gene by transgenic BAC rescue. *Cell* **89** (1997) 655-667.

[12]   A. Chawla and M.A. Lazar. Induction of Rev-ErbA alpha, an orphan receptor encoded on the opposite strand of the alpha-thyroid hormone receptor gene, during adipocyte differentiation. *J. Biol. Chem.* **268** (1993) 16265-16269.

[13]   B.M. Forman, J. Chen, B. Blumberg *et al.* Cross-talk among ROR alpha 1 and the Rev-erb family of orphan nuclear receptors. *Mol. Endocrinol.* **8** (1994) 1253-1261.

[14]   S.H. Munroe and M.A. Lazar. Inhibition of c-erbA mRNA splicing by a naturally occurring antisense RNA. *J. Biol. Chem.* **266** (1991) 22083-22086.

[15]   H. Onishi, S. Yamaguchi, K. Yagita *et al.* Rev-erbalpha gene expression in the mouse brain with special emphasis on its circadian profiles in the suprachiasmatic nucleus. *J. Neurosci. Res.* **68** (2002) 551-557.

[16]   I.P. Torra, V. Tsibulsky, F. Delaunay *et al.* Circadian and glucocorticoid regulation of Rev-erbalpha expression in liver. *Endocrinology* **141** (2000) 3799-3806.

[17]   A. Balsalobre, F. Damiola, U. Schibler. A serum shock induces circadian gene expression in mammalian tissue culture cells. *Cell* **93** (1998) 929-937. Comment in: *Cell* **93** (1998) 917-919.

[18]   S. Zvonic, A.A. Ptitsyn, S.A. Conrad *et al.* Characterization of peripheral circadian clocks in adipose tissues. *Diabetes* **55** (2006) 962-970.

[19]   J.P. Renaud, J.M. Harris, M. Downes *et al.* Structure-function analysis of the Rev-erbA and RVR ligand-binding domains reveals a large hydrophobic surface that mediates corepressor binding and a ligand cavity occupied by side chains. *Mol. Endocrinol.* **14** (2000) 700-717.

[20]   L. Yin, J. Wang, P.S. Klein *et al.* Nuclear receptor Rev-erbalpha is a critical lithium-sensitive component of the circadian clock. *Science* **311** (2006) 1002-1005.

[21]   H.P. Harding and M.A. Lazar. The monomer-binding orphan receptor Rev-Erb represses transcription as a dimer on a novel direct repeat. *Mol. Cell. Biol.* **15** (1995) 4791-4802. Erratum in: *Mol. Cell. Biol.* **15** (1995) 6479.

[22]   E. Raspe, G. Mautino, C. Duval *et al.* Transcriptional regulation of human Rev-erbalpha gene expression by the orphan nuclear receptor retinoic acid-related orphan receptor alpha. *J. Biol. Chem.* **277** (2002) 49275-49281.

[23]   G. Adelmant, A. Begue, D. Stehelin *et al.* A functional Rev-erb alpha responsive element located in the human Rev-erb alpha promoter mediates a repressing activity. *Proc. Natl. Acad. Sci. U.S.A.* **93** (1996) 3553-3558.

[24]   A.J. Lusis. Atherosclerosis. *Nature* **407** (2000) 233-241.

[25]   G.D. Barish, M. Downes, W.A. Alaynick *et al.* A Nuclear Receptor Atlas: macrophage activation. *Mol. Endocrinol.* **19** (2005) 2466-2477.

[26]   M. Teboul, M.A. Barrat-Petit, X.M. Li *et al.* Atypical patterns of circadian clock gene expression in human peripheral blood mononuclear cells. *J. Mol. Med.* **83** (2005) 693-699. Comment in: *J. Mol. Med.* **83** (2005) 655-656.

[27]   A. Dominguez-Rodriguez, P. Abreu-Gonzalez, M. Garcia *et al.* Light/dark patterns of interleukin-6 in relation to the pineal hormone melatonin in patients with acute myocardial infarction. *Cytokine* **26** (2004) 89-93.

[28]   P. Delerive, D. Monte, G. Dubois *et al.* The orphan nuclear receptor ROR alpha is a negative regulator of the inflammatory response. *EMBO Rep.* **2** (2001) 42-48.

[29]   S. Besnard, C. Heymes, R. Merval *et al.* Expression and regulation of the nuclear receptor RORalpha in human vascular cells. *FEBS Lett.* **511** (2002) 36-40.

[30]   H. Migita, N. Satozawa, J.H. Lin *et al.* RORalpha1 and RORalpha4 suppress TNF-alpha-induced VCAM-1 and ICAM-1 expression in human endothelial cells. *FEBS Lett.* **557** (2004) 269-274.

[31]   C. Hermann, S. von Aulock, O. Dehus *et al.* Endogenous cortisol determines the circadian rhythm of lipopolysaccharide-- but not lipoteichoic acid--inducible cytokine release. *Eur. J. Immunol.* **36** (2006) 371-379.

[32]   S. Koyanagi, S. Okazawa, Y. Kuramoto *et al.* Chronic treatment with prednisolone represses the circadian oscillation of clock gene expression in mouse peripheral tissues. *Mol. Endocrinol.* **20** (2006) 573-583.

[33]   F. Frédéric, C. Chianale, C. Oliver *et al.* Enhanced endocrine response to novel environment stress and lack of corticosterone circadian rhythm in staggerer (Rora sg/sg) mutant mice. *J. Neurosci. Res.* **83** (2006) 1525-1532.

[34]   T.K. Sato, S. Panda, L.J. Miraglia *et al.* A functional genomics strategy reveals Rora as a component of the mammalian circadian clock. *Neuron* **43** (2004) 527-537. Comment in: *Neuron* **43** (2004) 443-446.

[35]   F. Guillaumond, H. Dardente, V. Giguère *et al.* Differential control of Bmal1 circadian transcription by REV-ERB and ROR nuclear receptors. *J. Biol. Rhythms* **20** (2005) 391-403.

[36]   D.E. Vaughan. PAI-1 and atherothrombosis. *J. Thromb. Haemost.* **3** (2005) 1879-1883.

[37]   J. Wang, L. Yin, M.A. Lazar. The orphan nuclear receptor Rev-erb alpha regulates circadian expression of plasminogen activator inhibitor type 1. *J. Biol. Chem.* **281** (2006) 33842-33848.

[38]   U. Albrecht. Molecular orchestration of the hepatic circadian symphony. *Genome Biol.* **7** (2006) 234.

[39]   H. Ando, H. Yanagihara, Y. Hayashi *et al.* Rhythmic messenger ribonucleic acid expression of clock genes and adipocytokines in mouse visceral adipose tissue. *Endocrinology* **146** (2005) 5631-5636.

[40]   G. Block. Keep time, stay healthy. *Sci. Aging Knowledge Environ.* **2005** (2005) pe13.

[41]   F.W. Turek, C. Joshu, A. Kohsaka *et al.* Obesity and metabolic syndrome in circadian Clock mutant mice. *Science* **308** (2005) 1043-1045.

[42]   D.L. Williams and M.W. Schwartz. Out of synch: Clock mutation causes obesity in mice. *Cell Metab.* **1** (2005) 355-356.

[43]   R.D. Rudic, P. McNamara, A.M. Curtis *et al.* BMAL1 and CLOCK, two essential components of the circadian clock, are involved in glucose homeostasis. *PLoS Biol.* **2** (2004) e377.

[44]   E. Raspe, H. Duez, P. Gervois *et al.* Transcriptional regulation of apolipoprotein C-III gene expression by the orphan nuclear receptor RORalpha. *J. Biol. Chem.* **276** (2001) 2865-2871.

[45]   N. Vu-Dac, S. Chopin-Delannoy, P. Gervois *et al.* The nuclear receptors peroxisome proliferator-activated receptor alpha and Rev-erbalpha mediate the species-specific regulation of apolipoprotein A-I expression by fibrates. *J. Biol. Chem.* **273** (1998) 25713-25720.

[46]   N. Vu-Dac, P. Gervois, T. Grotzinger *et al.* Transcriptional regulation of apolipoprotein A-I gene expression by the nuclear receptor RORalpha. *J. Biol. Chem.* **272** (1997) 22401-22404.

[47]   W.A. Boisvert, A.S. Black, L.K. Curtiss. ApoA1 reduces free cholesterol accumulation in atherosclerotic lesions of ApoE-deficient mice transplanted with ApoE-expressing macrophages. *Arterioscler. Thromb. Vasc. Biol.* **19** (1999) 525-530.

[48]   P. Gervois, S. Chopin-Delannoy, A. Fadel *et al.* Fibrates increase human REV-ERBalpha expression in liver via a novel peroxisome proliferator-activated receptor response element. *Mol. Endocrinol.* **13** (1999) 400-409.

[49]   A. Kassam, J.P. Capone, R.A. Rachubinski. Orphan nuclear hormone receptor RevErbalpha modulates expression from the promoter of the hydratase-dehydrogenase gene by inhibiting peroxisome proliferator-activated receptor alpha-dependent transactivation. *J. Biol. Chem.* **274** (1999) 22895-22900.

[50]   M.H. Hsu, C.N. Palmer, W. Song *et al.* A carboxyl-terminal extension of the zinc finger domain contributes to the specificity and polarity of peroxisome proliferator-activated receptor DNA binding. *J. Biol. Chem.* **273** (1998) 27988-27997.

[51]   R.A. Derlacz, P. Poplawski, M. Napierala *et al.* Melatonin-induced modulation of glucose metabolism in primary cultures of rabbit kidney-cortex tubules. *J. Pineal Res.* **38** (2005) 164-169.

[52]   K. Winiarska, T. Fraczyk, D. Malinska *et al.* Melatonin attenuates diabetes-induced oxidative stress in rabbits. *J. Pineal Res.* **40** (2006) 168-176.

[53]   E. Grossman, M. Laudon, R. Yalcin *et al.* Melatonin reduces night blood pressure in patients with nocturnal hypertension. *Am. J. Med.* **119** (2006) 898-902.

[54]   P. Pevet, L. Agez, B. Bothorel *et al.* Melatonin in the multi-oscillatory mammalian circadian world. *Chronobiol. Int.* **23** (2006) 39-51.

[55]   I. Wiesenberg, M. Missbach, C. Carlberg. The potential role of the transcription factor RZR/ROR as a mediator of nuclear melatonin signaling. *Restor. Neurol. Neurosci.* **12** (1998) 143-150.

Nuclear Receptors as Molecular Targets for Cardiometabolic and Central Nervous System Diseases
J.L. Junien and B. Staels (Eds.)
IOS Press, 2008

Author Index